Handbook of
Fracture
Classifications

Handbook of
Fracture
Classifications

Mukul Mohindra
MS (Ortho), DNB, MNAMS, Dip. SICOT (Belgium), FNB
(Arthroscopy and Sports Medicine)
Specialist Orthopedics, CGHS Wing
Central Institute of Orthopedics
Safdarjung Hospital and VMM College
New Delhi

Anish Agarwalla
MBBS, MS (Ortho)
Central Institute of Orthopedics
Safdarjung Hospital and VMM College
New Delhi

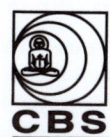

CBS Publishers & Distributors Pvt Ltd

New Delhi • Bengaluru • Chennai • Kochi • Kolkata • Mumbai
Hyderabad • Jharkhand • Nagpur • Patna • Pune • Uttarakhand

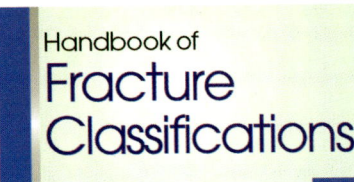

ISBN: 978-93-86478-41-2

Copyright © Authors and Publisher

First Edition 2017

Published by Satish Kumar Jain and Produced by Varun Jain for

CBS Publishers & Distributors Pvt Ltd

4819/XI Prahlad Street, 24 Ansari Road, Daryaganj, New Delhi 110 002, India.
Ph: 23289259, 23266861, 23266867   Fax: 011-23243014   Website: www.cbspd.com
e-mail: delhi@cbspd.com; cbspubs@airtelmail.in.

Corporate Office: 204 FIE, Industrial Area, Patparganj, Delhi 110 092, India
Ph: 4934 4934   Fax: 4934 4935   e-mail: publishing@cbspd.com; publicity@cbspd.com

Branches

- **Bengaluru:** Seema House 2975, 17th Cross, K.R. Road,
  Banasankari 2nd Stage, Bengaluru 560 070, Karnataka, India
  Ph: +91-80-26771678/79   Fax: +91-80-26771680   e-mail: bangalore@cbspd.com
- **Chennai:** 7, Subbaraya Street, Shenoy Nagar, Chennai 600 030, Tamil Nadu, India
  Ph: +91-44-26260666, 26208620   Fax: +91-44-42032115   e-mail: chennai@cbspd.com
- **Kochi:** Ashana House, No. 39/1904, AM Thomas Road, Valanjambalam, Eranakulam 682 018, Kochi, Kerala, India
  Ph: +91-484-4059061-65   Fax: +91-484-4059065   e-mail: kochi@cbspd.com
- **Kolkata:** No. 6/B, Ground Floor, Rameswar Shaw Road, Kolkata-700014 (West Bengal), India
  Ph: +91-33-2289-1126, 2289-1127, 2289-1128   e-mail: kolkata@cbspd.com
- **Mumbai:** 83-C, Dr E Moses Road, Worli, Mumbai-400018, Maharashtra, India
  Ph: +91-22-24902340/41   Fax: +91-22-24902342   e-mail: mumbai@cbspd.com

Representatives

- **Hyderabad**   0-9885175004
- **Patna**   0-9334159340
- **Jharkhand**   0-9811541605
- **Pune**   0-9623451994
- **Nagpur**   0-9021734563
- **Uttarakhand**   0-9716462459

Printed at International Print-o-Pac Ltd. India

to

my parents for their blessings
my wife Bhumika for her unconditional love and my family for always being there

Mukul Mohindra

my parents Mr. Banwarilal Agarwalla and Smt. Sarita Agarwalla, whose nurturing gave me courage to dream, my sister Nikita who strengthened me to realize my dreams and my brother Aman who has always been there whenever I needed support.

Anish Agarwalla

Foreword

Orthopedics is a vast subject and fracture classification is an indispensable part of it. Its very important for the young generation to be acquainted with the same. But there is a lack of literature dealing with fracture classification. Teaching methodology and orthopedics course curriculum have undergone plethora of changes in the past decade.

Handbook of Fracture Classifications by Dr Anish and Dr Mukul has narratively and comprehensively explained the basic concepts and types of fracture classification which the orthopedic students must know. The inclusion of excellent colored diagrams, 3D pictures and table depictions are highly informative, with an eye on daily orthopedic practice dealing.

Having gone through a few chapters, I am fully convinced that this book with its clarity yet in-depth elaboration of orthopedic classification will be an asset to every orthopedic student.

Dr Mukul and Dr Anish have worked with me at Central Institute of Orthopedics, VMM College and Safdarjung Hospital and have an amazing clarity of clinical foundations of orthopedics. I strongly feel this book is a must on the shelf of every student of orthopedics. I am sure the authors will further justify every subsequent edition, keeping in mind the fast changing orthopedic technology. I wish the book and the authors all the success in furthering the knowledge of orthopedics among the students.

Ramesh Kumar
Director Professor
Director, Central Institute of Orthopaedics
VMMC and Safdarjung Hospital
New Delhi

Foreword

It gives me immense pleasure to write the foreword to *Handbook of Fracture Classifications* written by Anish Agarwalla and Mukul Mohindra. I believe that this book will fill the lacunae in undergraduate and postgraduate teaching. Fracture classification is a diverse topic and this book covers all the fracture classification in orthopedics in simple language with excellent illustrations. First time, I see a book which shows all the classifications in orthopedics being clearly illustrated in figures and tables, with 3D illustration. Important table and figures in color, makes reading easy, matter easy to remember and has high recall value. It also includes AO classification in a detailed and simple manner.

Both Anish and Mukul have a flair for teaching and its appropriate that they have come up with this excellent book. I hope that all the undergraduates and postgraduates will find it useful and start practising writing classification in their pescription. I wish the authors and the book success in enlightening all of us.

LG Krishna
Director Professor
Central Institute of Orthopedics
VMMC and Safdarjung Hospital
New Delhi

Contributors

Anurag Gupta MS (Ortho)
Central Institute of Orthopedics
Safdarjung Hospital and VMM College, New Delhi
Spine fractures classifications

Gaurav Saini
Associate Consultant
Fortis Hospital, Mohali
For helping with acetabular fracture images

Preface

Medical fraternity commonly comes across fractures in trauma services as well as OPD settings making, it important to identify all the fractures and grade them according to severity foundation for providing the best management and rehabilitation.

Orthopedicians while dealing with fracture patients need to evaluate, classify and grade the fractures according to the universal classification, so that anyone attending the patient after the primary surgeon can understand the severity and hence a better management is offered. Any deviation from standard grading leads to chaos.

The idea of writing a book on fracture classification came to the authors in the early years of residency upon facing difficulty in dealing with classifications and lack of compilation of the vast literature for the same. Thus we took up this herculean task of reviewing the literature, compiling and sequencing various classifications of fracture, in this book making the understanding, memorising and application of the same simpler. They started working on this book and updated all classifications. The real attraction are the three-dimensional images especially of pelvic fractures which includes special 3D virtual CT images used lately for computer aided surgery. Pediatric fractures, AO classifications are also discussed in detail and in a simplified manner to enhance understanding and recall.

'And all is in the well when end is in the well', a quote that needs no description. So to ensure the end is not in a well, we have included fracture eponyms with fancy names. As new classifications keep on evolving, its important to keep oneself updated, a part thoroughly kept in mind while writing the book.

And to sum up, we believe that "we don't have the right to complain when we ourselves walk imperfectly" …. Thus this book has been written to give readers a perfect mentor and a "all in one book" for their daily practice. Readers are requested to contact authors in case they find any mistakes.

Mukul Mohindra

Anish Agarwalla
dranishagarwalla@gmail.com
Delhi, June 2017

Acknowledgements

This book was a dream project for both of us but efforts of a number of people stand behind the stage. Without them the dream would have never come true. It is our pleasure to acknowledge their efforts as their support formed that pillar of strength that helped us finish this herculean task with such an ease.

The seeds of this book were sown in Central Institute of Orthopaedics, VMMC and Safdarjung Hospital. It was the vision of our Director, Dr Ramesh Kumar, to motivate us to begin this journey. His visionary leadership is an encouragement to every young budding orthopod. Problems unfolded as we travelled the path but the guidance and blessings by our teachers Dr LG Krishna and Dr RK Chopra helped us pave our way through. Their vast experience and sea of knowledge helped us at every single step. Dr Naval Bhatia, Dr Vikas Gupta, Dr BP Sharma and Dr Davinder were all a source of motivation whenever we got into any dilemma. The friendly nature of Dr Narendra Kumar, Dr Hitesh Lal, Dr Jatin Talwar, Dr Tankeswar Baruah, Dr RK Beniwal, Dr Ashish Rustagi, Dr Prateek Behera and Dr Sandeep Shaina helped us to clear many doubts and we could ring them at any time for any assistance.

I (Dr Anish) would be grateful to goddess Saraswati and Shiva for catering me good mental and physical health that made timely completion of this book possible. I would take this pleasure to thank my teachers whom I owe what I am today. My alma mater Gauhati Medical College, Guwahati and its orthopedics department under Dr Tulsi Bhattacharjee are the reason I took orthopedics. The Central Institute of Orthopaedics, VMMC and Safdarjung Hospital carved a stone into a structure which had a meaning. I am short of words to thank my guide Prof Dr LG Krishna (Director Professor) who was not just my guide but my mentor and guardian both academically and personally. I have immense respect for Dr RK Chopra (Director Professor) who always behaves as a fatherly figure to his juniors and encourages them to achieve heights in their life. I would like to remember my senior residents Dr Akshat Sharma, Dr Ketan Pandey, Dr Kavish, Dr Abhimanyu, Dr Tejasvi, Dr Sandeep, Dr Sahu, Dr Amit and Dr Abhishek Vaish who always encouraged me and gave me free time out of busy duty schedule, so that I could complete the book in time. Dr Sathyamurthy, Dr Narendran P, Dr Hemendra, Dr Vikash Moond have always been source of inspiration. I would be failing in my duty if I don't thank my friend Dr Anurag Gupta and Dr Tarun Verma for helping me in the book and Dr Saloni Gupta and Dr Anamika Thakral for igniting that spark in me for writing the book. I would also extend my thanks to my motivator cum my guide Dr Mukul Mohindra for encouraging the idea of this book and being an equal and indispensable part of this journey.

I (Dr Mukul) would like to first thank my teachers whom I owe a lot. Dr M Yamin (Director Professor, DMC and H, Ludhiana) has been a mentor to whom I have always looked up. Dr Daljeet Singh, Dr Sandeep Puri and Dr Rajoo Singh have been the role models I aspire to be. The support and encouragement I received from Dr Hemlata Badyal, Dr Lily Walia, Dr Hitant Vohra, Dr Jagjiv Sharma, Dr Deepinder Chinna, Dr Sarit, Dr Harpreet Puri, Dr Poonam Singh, Dr Sunil Juneja, Dr Rajneesh Garg, Dr Alka Dogra and Dr Bajwa sculpted in me the confidence to face the challenges of life. I find myself short of words when it comes to thank my guide in postgraduation, Prof Dr SS Sangwan (Former Vice Chancellor, University of Health Sciences, Rohtak). The skills I have today to a great extent belong to Dr RC Siwach, Dr NK Magu, Dr RK Gupta, Dr Roop Singh, Dr ZS Kundu, Dr A Devgun, Dr R Rohilla, Dr Pradeep Kamboj, my teachers during my PG. I would be failing in my duty if I don't thank my teachers at Maulana Azad Medical College, Dr A Dhal, Dr AK Gupta, Dr VK Gautam, Dr Lalit Maini, Dr Vinod Kumar, Dr Manoj, Dr Sumit Sural and Dr Dhananjay Sabat who made me the person I am today. My job would be incomplete without extending my thanks to Dr Deepak Chaudhary, a great motivator whose blessings infused in me the confidence to begin this journey. Problems unfolded as I travelled the path but the guidance by my teachers Dr Himanshu Kataria, Dr Deepak Joshi and Dr Vineet Jain helped me pave through. Dr Ankit Goyal, Dr Nitin Mehta, Dr Pallav Mishra, Dr Himanshu Gupta, Dr Ajay Lal, Dr Vivek Shankar and Dr Ashutosh Jha were all a source of motivation. Never can I miss Dr George Maceras who made my training in Greece during my fellowship a memorable one. A special thanks to Dr SP Singh and Dr Shyama Gupta, Dr Anurag Jain and Dr Pandey, Dr BP Sharma, Dr Beniwal and Dr Sandeep Shaina for giving me the space to grow. And last but no way the least, support by my seniors, colleagues, juniors and friends was indispensable. Dr Jitesh Jain, Dr Navdeep, Dr Ashwani Singh, Dr Naveen MG, Dr Lalait Bafna, Dr Mohd. Shafi Bhat, Dr Darsh Goyal, Dr Milind Tanwar, Dr Rahul, Dr Manoj Arya, Dr Shiv Chouksey, Dr Rakesh Daripa, Dr Himanshu Bhargava, Dr Brahma Prakash, Dr Pawan Sharma, Dr Utkarsh, Dr Atul Mahajan, Dr Pankaj, Dr Sunny, Dr Dickey, Dr Chandan Jasrotia, Dr Rohit, Dr Rishav Gupta, Dr Sanjay Arora, Dr Gaurav Saini and Dr Ankit Ruhella, thank you all for being there. I would also extend my thanks to my motivators come my teachers Dr Sumer Sethi, Dr Tushar Mehta, Dr Pritish Singh and Dr Kamal Bali.

The contributors of this book deserve special thanks for the valuable time they devoted and the immense hard work and energy they had put in. Despite their busy schedules, even at a single call they stood by us to write the chapters comprehensively. Guys this project never would have been an accomplishment without your efforts.

Finally, we would like to thank CBS Publishers and the team of Mr YN Arjuna, the real men behind the stage. Their tiring efforts turned this dream of ours into a reality. We would be looking forward to work more with the wonderful team in coming future.

Mukul Mohindra

Anish Agarwalla

Contents

Foreword *by* Ramesh Kumar   *vii*

Foreword *by* LG Krishna   *ix*

Contributors   *xi*

Preface   *xiii*

1. AO Classification of Fractures (Müller's AO/OTA Classification)   1

2. Open and Closed Fractures   18

3. Shoulder and Upper Limb   23

4. Pelvis and Lower Limb   52

5. Spine   92

6. Pediatric Injuries   108

7. Periprosthetic Fractures   126

8. Fracture Eponyms   132

Index   135

AO Classification of Fractures (Müller's AO/OTA Classification)

In orthopaedics, fractures are classified in various ways. Historically they were named after the physician who first described the fracture conditions, however, now there are more systematic classifications in place currently.

Fractures can be classified according to the following ways. For examples:

1. Nature of trauma—closed/open
2. Nature of mechanism—traumatic/pathological
3. Displaced/undisplaced
4. According to site/bone involved
5. Fracture pattern—simple/comminuted
6. Named on authors—Frykman, Cotton, Neer, etc.

Thus adding complexity to classification system.

"AO" is an initialism for the German "Arbeitsgemeinschaft für Osteosynthesefragen", the predecessor of the AO Foundation. In 1984, a group of AO surgeons led by Maurice E Müller published the "Classification of Fractures", which was the first comprehensive, systematic fracture classification system. While it has been referred to by many different names, it was officially named the "Müller AO classification of fractures—long bones". It fulfilled a long-felt need for a universally applicable and acceptable classification system. Later, this initial system was further developed by a joint group of surgeons and researchers of the AO and of the American Orthopaedic Trauma Association (OTA) and is now officially known as the "AO/OTA classification of fractures and dislocations".

This is a unique and comprehensive classification published initially by AO foundation, which can be applied to fracture of all bones. It is an alphanumerical classification, i.e. numbers and alphabets are used to classify a fracture which allows fracture patterns to be given a digital platform. Recently a pediatric version has also been published.

Different authors may classify same fracture differently, as multiple classifications are described for same fracture, which makes following fracture scoring/treatment/prognosis/guideline for management difficult in research paper. There is always a lack of consensus, among authors to follow a single classification, as all have some advantages and disadvantages. However, AO classification negates this effect by a 5-element alphanumeric code in fracture classification with each element describing the following (Table 1.1) parts, thus allowing a uniform classification to each and every bones in human body. Because of this uniformity fracture classification can be used in a digitalised platform and can be followed in all research papers to allow authors a common albeit complex classification.

TABLE 1.1

Localisation		Morphology		
Bone	Segment	Type	Group	Subgroup
1/2/3/4	1/2/3/(4)	A/B/C	1/2/3	.1/.2/.3

LOCALISATION

First, each fracture is assigned with 2 numbers which denotes the bone it affects and the 2nd digit to indicate the part of bone involved in fracture. Each major bone is given a number (Fig. 1.2) like humerus, forearm bones, the femur and leg bones have been assigned 1, 2, 3 and 4 respectively and each long bone is divided into three segments; proximal segment, diaphysis and distal segment, which are assigned 1, 2 and 3 numbers respectively (Fig. 1.1 and Table 1.2).

TYPE

Definition of Fracture Subtypes

- *Extra-articular.* Fracture does not involve the articular surface but may be within the capsule of the joint. They include apophyseal and metaphyseal fractures.
- *Articular, partial.* Only part of the joint is involved while the remainder remains attached to the diaphysis.
- *Articular, complete.* The joint surface is fractured and the entire joint surface is separated from the diaphysis. The severity of these fractures depends on whether their articular and metaphyseal components are simple or multifragmentary.
- *Impacted.* A fracture in which the opposing bone surfaces are driven into each other and

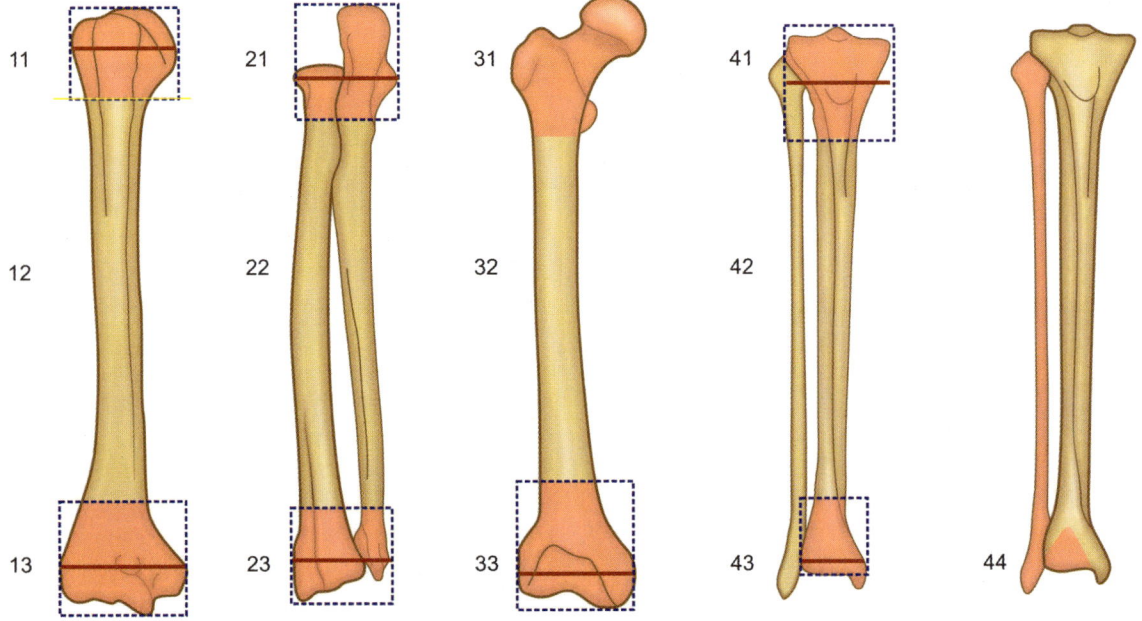

Fig. 1.1: Assigning number for the segment of long bone involved (c.f. malleoli in tibia and fibula are considered separately under segment categorization and assigned number-4).

TABLE 1.2

	1	2	3	4
Bone	Humerus	Radius and ulna	Femur	Tibia and fibula
Segment	Proximal segment	Diaphyseal segment	Distal segment	Malleolar segment (only used with tibia and fibula

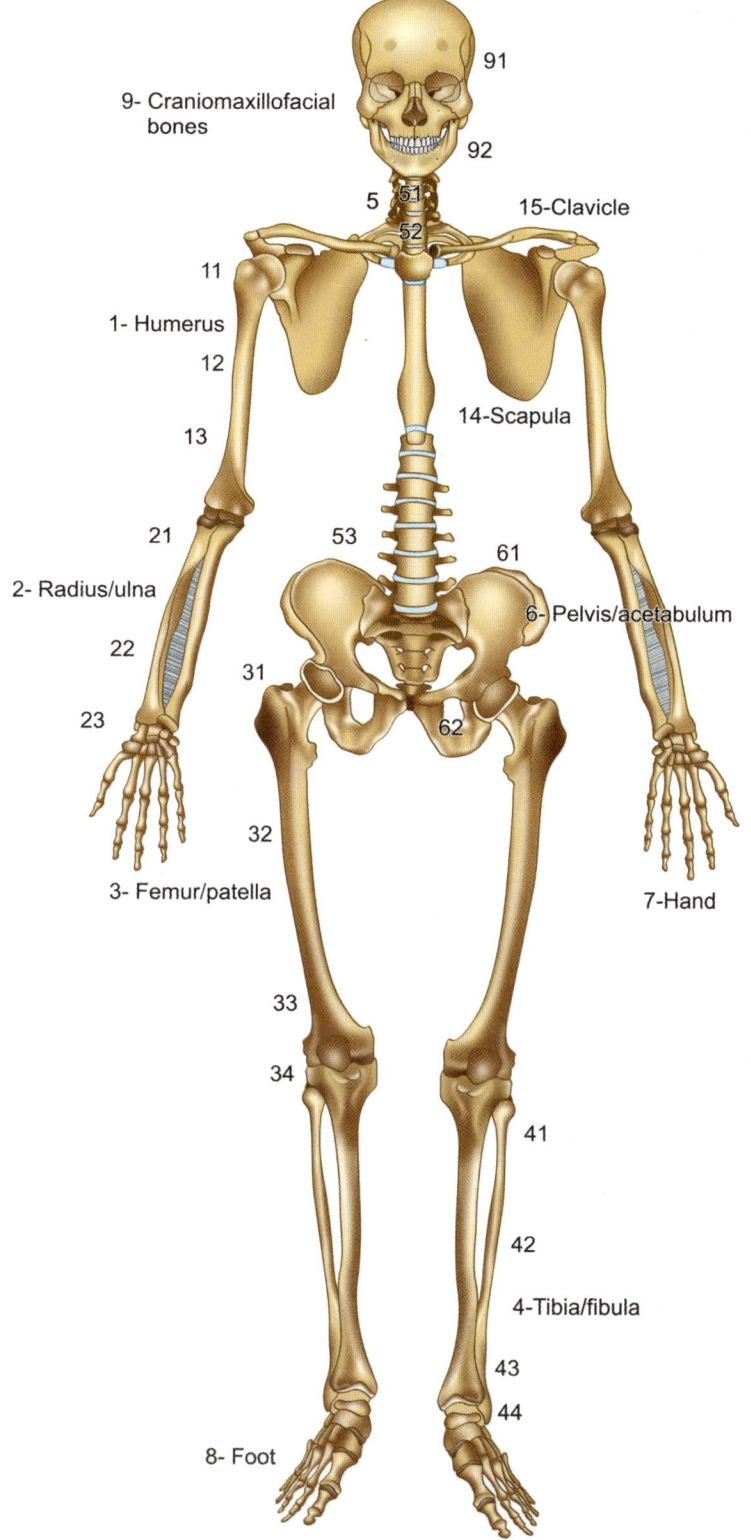

Fig. 1.2: AO classification: Each major bone is assigned a number (1–9).

behave as a single unit. This is a combined clinical and radiological diagnosis.

- **Simple.** There is a single fracture line producing two fracture fragments. Simple fractures of the diaphysis or metaphysis are spiral, oblique, or transverse.
- **Multi-fragmentary.** A fracture with more than one fracture line so that there are three or more pieces. It includes wedge and complex fractures.
- **Complex.** Fracture with one or more intermediate fragment(s) in which there is no contact between the main fragments after reduction. The complex fractures are spiral, segmental, or irregular.
- **Wedge.** Fracture complex with a third fragment in which, after reduction, there is some direct contact between the two main fragments.

- **Pure split.** An articular fracture in which there is a longitudinal metaphyseal and articular split, without any additional osteochondral lesion.
- **Pure depression.** An articular fracture in which there is only a depression of the articular surface without a split. The depression may be central or peripheral.
- **Multi-fragmentary depression.** A fracture in which part of the joint is depressed and the fragments are completely separated.

Fracture sustained by concerned segment is further given an alphabetic categorization from A to C depending upon the fracture pattern (Fig. 1.3 and Table 1.3).

Following are the exceptions to the above step (Table 1.4).

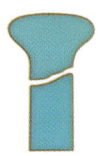

Extra-articular
Articular surface not involved

Simple
Only for fracture line, with cortical contact exceeding 90% after reduction

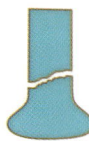

Extra-articular
Articular surface not involved

Partial articular
One part articular surface involved, other part remain attached to main bone

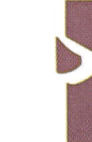

Wedge
A total of ≥3 fragments, with main fragments having contact after reduction

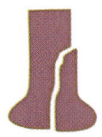

Partial articular
One part of articular surface involved, other part remain attached to main bone

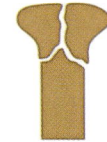

Complete articular
Articular surface completely detached from the main bone

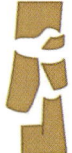

Complex
≥3 fragments, with main fragments having no contact after reduction

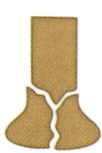

Complete articular
Articular surface completely detached from the main bone

Fig. 1.3: AO classification: Assigning alphabet to fracture pattern of the involved segment.

TABLE 1.3

Segment	A	B	C
1	Extra-articular	Partial articular	Complete articular
2	Simple	Wedge	Complex
3	Extra-articular	Partial articular	Complete articular

TABLE 1.4

Localisation	A	B	C
11: Proximal humerus	Extra-articular, unifocal	Extra-articular, bifocal	Articular
31: Proximal femur	Extra-articular, trochanteric	Extra-articular, neck	Articular, head
44: Malleoli	Infrasyndesmotic	Transyndesmotic	Suprasyndesmotic

GROUPS AND SUBGROUPS

Till now, we have described classification according to the bone, part of the bone involved and fracture line. Now the fracture is given 2 further numbers to denote the fracture pattern and geometry (Fig. 1.4 and Table 1.5).

For segment 1 and 3 (epiphyseal and metaphyseal) fractures (Table 1.6 and Fig. 1.5).

Subgroups are then used to describe the fractures in terms of displacement (versus apposition, which is the degree to which the parts are in contact with each other), rotation, angulation and shortening.

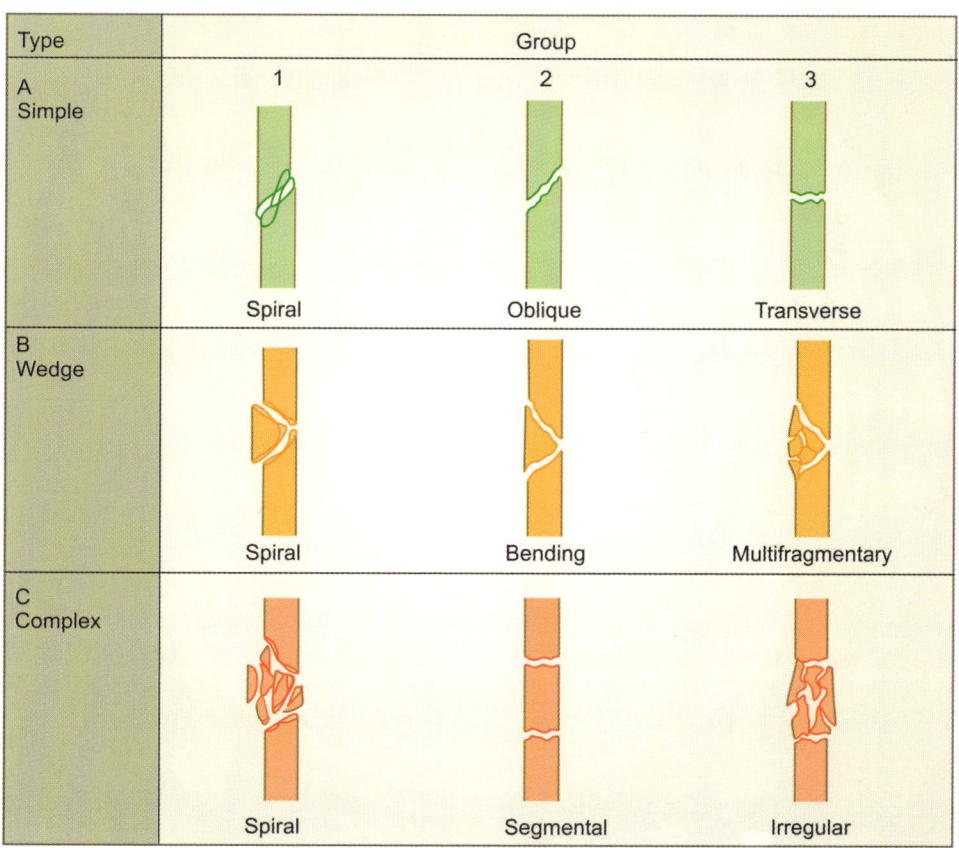

Fig. 1.4: AO A/B/C—1/2/3 sub-types.

TABLE 1.5

Type	Group		
	1	*2*	*3*
A: Simple	Spiral	Oblique	Transverse
B: Wedge	Spiral	Bending	Multifragmentary
C: Complex	Spiral	Segmental	Irregular

TABLE 1.6

Type	Group		
	1	*2*	*3*
A: Extra-articular	Simple	Wedge	Complex
B: Partial articular	Split (tibia)/lateral condyle (distal humerus/distal femur)	Depression (tibia)/medial condyle (distal humerus/distal femur)	Split-depression (tibia)/coronal (distal humerus/distal femur)
C: Articular	Simple articular, simple metaphyseal	Simple articular, complex metaphyseal	Complex articular, complex metaphyseal

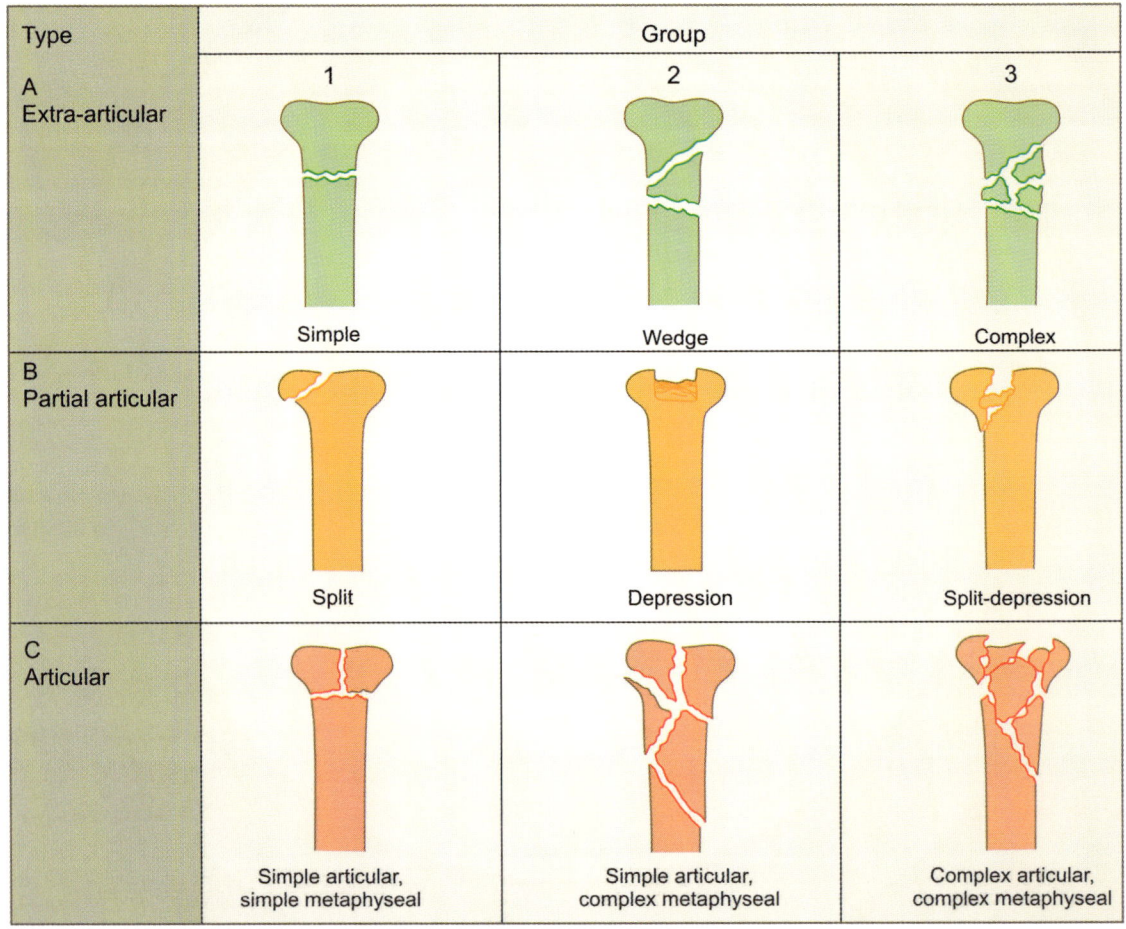

Fig. 1.5: AO epiphyseal and metaphyseal fractures.

AO PEDIATRIC COMPREHENSIVE CLASSIFICATION OF LONG BONE FRACTURES

A pediatric version of the long-bone classification was published in 2006 (Table 1.7, Figs 1.6 and 1.7) to further classify fractures of immature bone and so the effects on future growth.

TABLE 1.7

	Localisation			Morphology	
Bone	Segment	Type	Child	Severity	Exceptions
1/2/3/4	1/2/3	E/M/D	1–9	.1/.2	I–IV

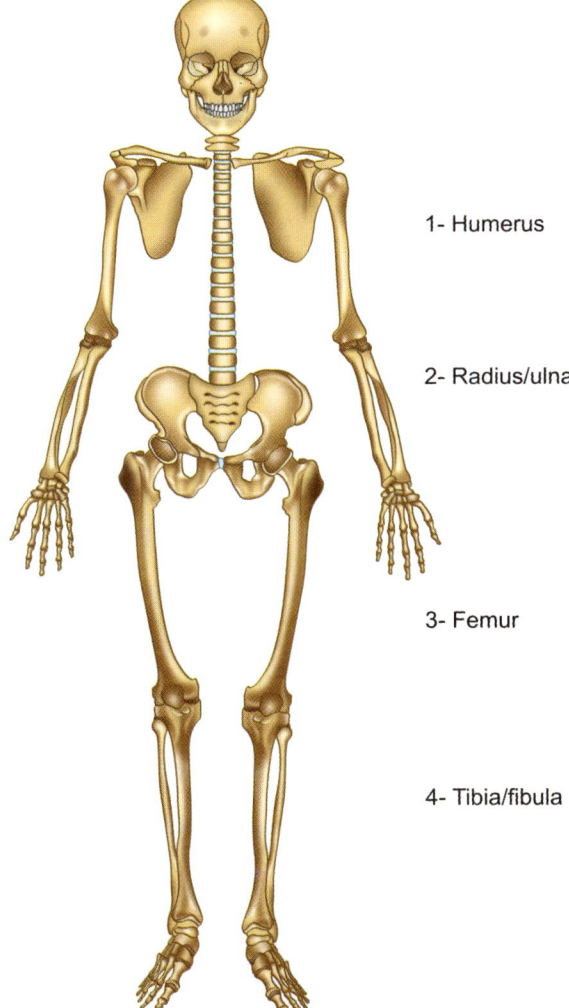

1- Humerus

2- Radius/ulna

3- Femur

4- Tibia/fibula

Fig. 1.6: Schematic diagram to denote bone numerology

EXTENDED AO NUMERIC SYSTEM FOR OTHER BONES

TABLE 1.8

Localisation		Region/Bone
Bone	**Segment**	
1	4	Scapula
	5	Clavicle
3	4	Patella
5	1	Cervical spine
	2	Thoracic spine
	3	Lumbar spine
6	1	Pelvic ring
	2	Acetabulum
7	1	Lunate
	2	Scaphoid
	3	Capitate
	4	Hamate
	5	Triquetrum and pisiform
	6	Trapezium and trapezoid
	7	Metacarpus
	8	Phalanges
	9	Multiple fractures
8	1	Talus
	2	Calcaneus
	3	Navicular
	4	Cuboid
	5	Cuneiforms
	7	Metatarsus
	8	Phalanges
	9	Multiple fractures
9	1	Cranio-midfacial
	2	Mandible

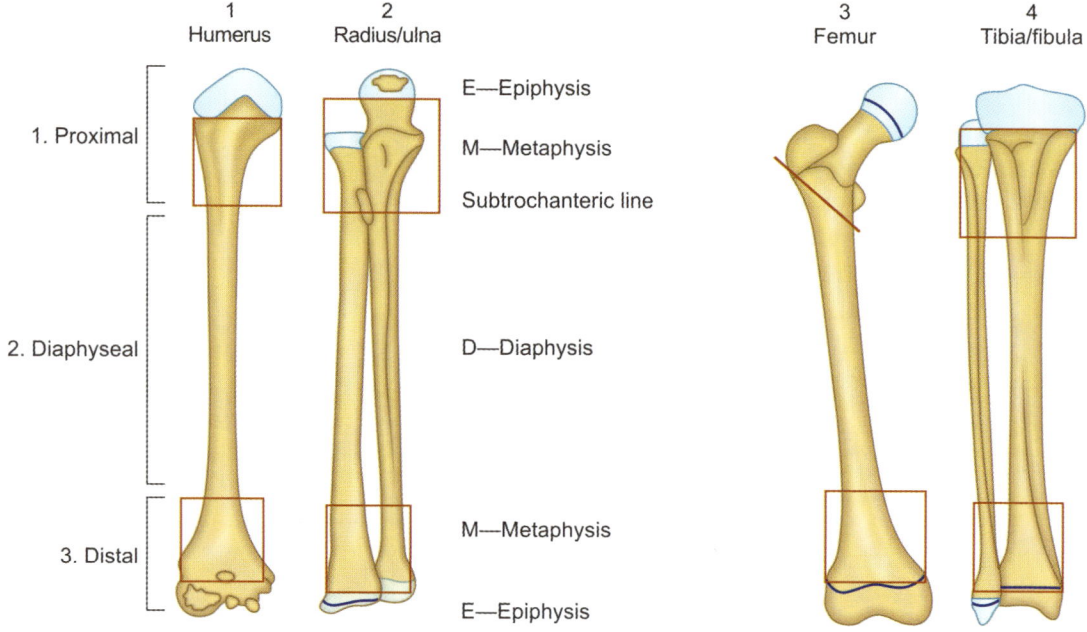

Fig. 1.7: Schematic diagrams show bone segment and parts involved

AO CLASSIFICATION OF INDIVIDUAL BONES

1. Humerus

11. Proximal (Fig. 1.8a)

11-A	**extra-articular unifocal fracture**
11-A1	tuberosity
11-A2	impacted metaphyseal
11-A3	nonimpacted metaphyseal
11-B	**extra-articular bifocal fracture**
11-B1	with metaphyseal impaction
11-B2	without metaphyseal impaction
11-B3	with glenohumeral dislocation
11-C	**articular fracture**
11-C1	with slight displacement
11-C2	impacted with marked displacement
11-C3	dislocated

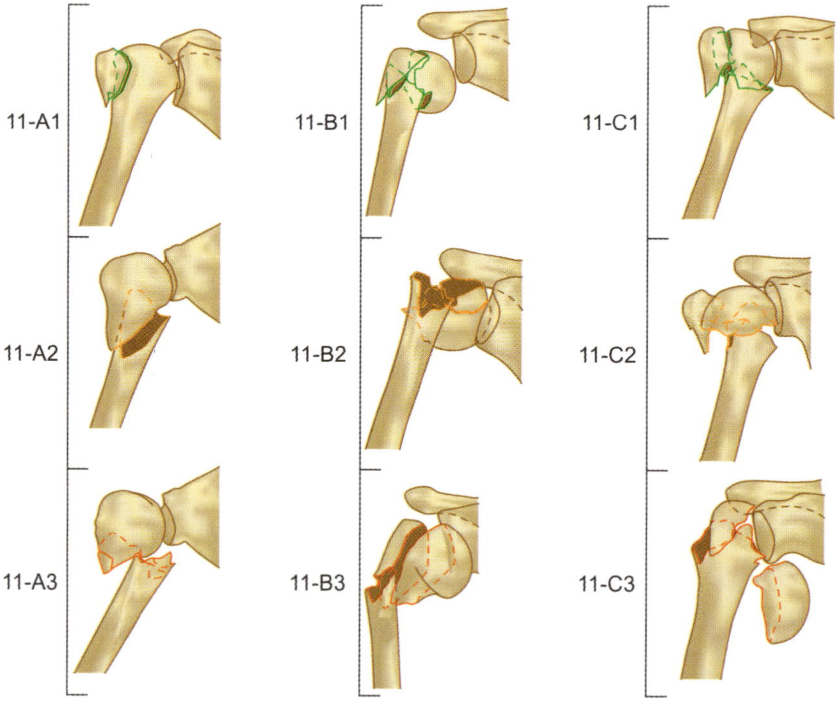

11-A1   11-B1   11-C1

11-A2   11-B2   11-C2

11-A3   11-B3   11-C3

Fig. 1.8a

12. *Diaphyseal* (Fig. 1.8b)

12-A	simple fracture
12-A1	spiral
12-A2	oblique (> 30°)
12-A3	transverse (< 30°)

12-B	wedge fracture
12-B1	spiral wedge
12-B2	bending wedge
12-B3	fragmented wedge

12-C	complex fracture
12-C1	spiral
12-C2	segmental
12-C3	irregular

Fig. 1.8b

13. *Distal* (Fig. 1.8c)

13-A	extra-articular fracture
13-A1	apophyseal avulsion
13-A2	metaphyseal simple
13-A3	metaphyseal multifragmentary

13-B	partial articular fracture
13-B1	sagittal lateral condyle
13-B2	sagittal medial condyle
13-B3	coronal

13-C	complete articular fracture
13-C1	articular simple, metaphyseal simple
13-C2	articular simple, metaphyseal multifragmentary
13-C3	articular multifragmentary

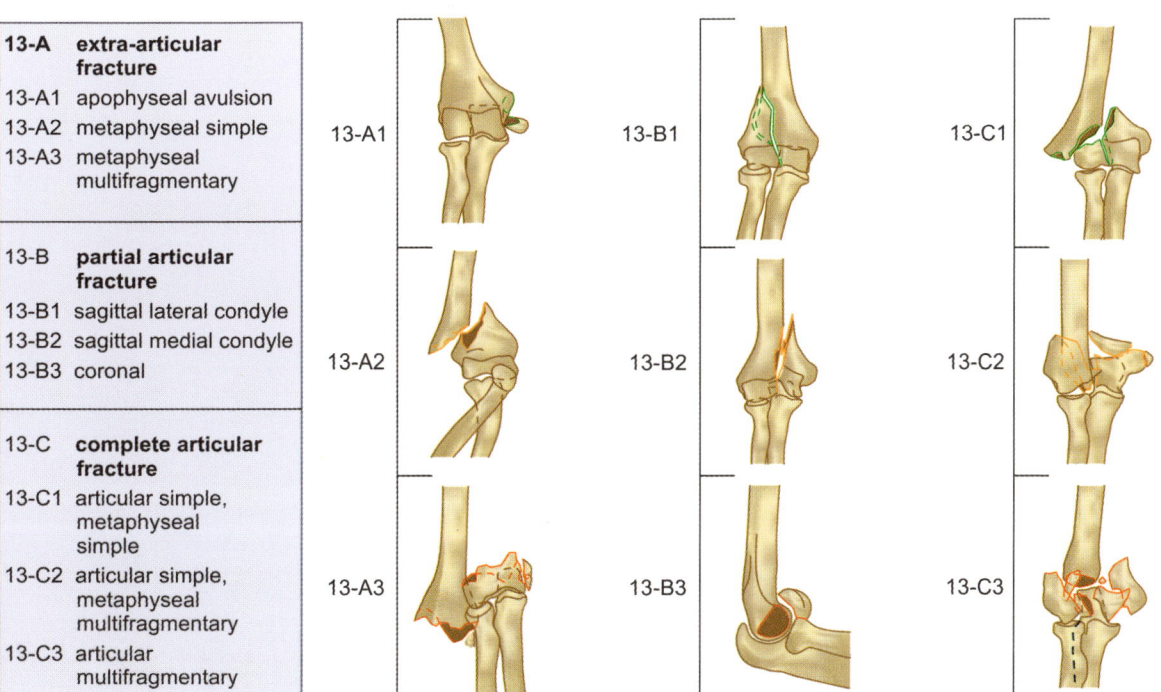

Fig. 1.8c

2. Radius

21. *Proximal* (Fig. 1.9a)

21-A	extra-articular fracture
21-A1	ulna fractured, radius intact
21-A2	radius fractured, ulna intact
21-A3	both bones

21-B	articular fracture
21-B1	ulna fractured, radius intact
21-B2	radius fractured, ulna intact
21-B3	one bone articular fracture, other extra-articular

21-C	articular fracture of both bones
21-C1	simple
21-C2	one articular fracture simple, other articular fracture multifragmentary
21-C3	multifragmentary

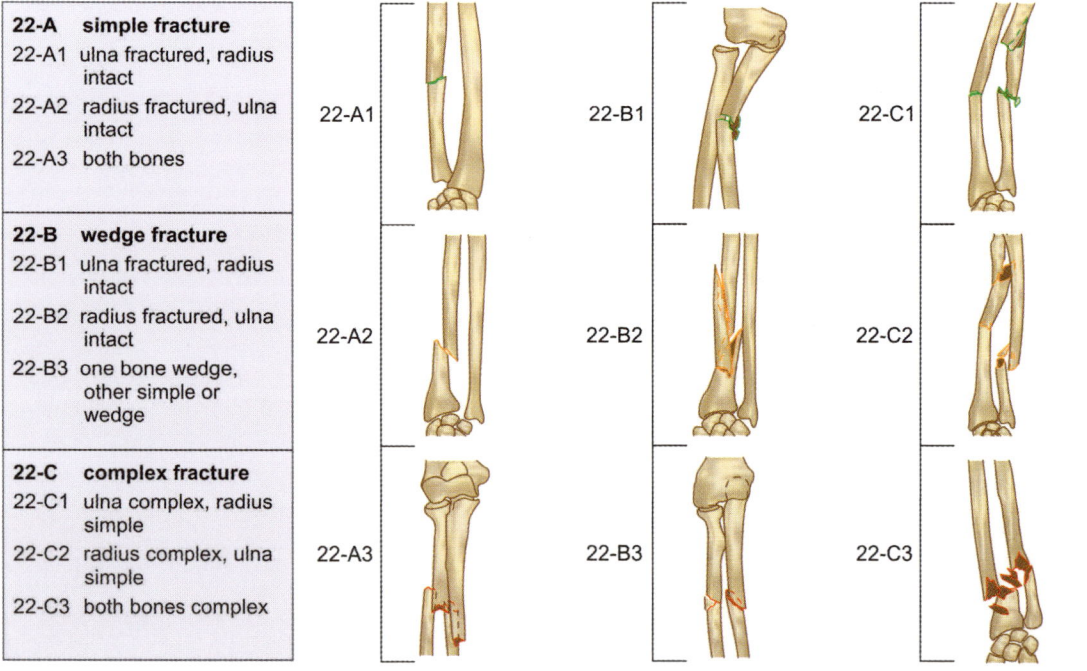

Fig. 1.9a

22. *Diaphyseal* (Fig. 1.9b)

22-A	simple fracture
22-A1	ulna fractured, radius intact
22-A2	radius fractured, ulna intact
22-A3	both bones

22-B	wedge fracture
22-B1	ulna fractured, radius intact
22-B2	radius fractured, ulna intact
22-B3	one bone wedge, other simple or wedge

22-C	complex fracture
22-C1	ulna complex, radius simple
22-C2	radius complex, ulna simple
22-C3	both bones complex

Fig. 1.9b

23. *Distal* (Fig. 1.9c)

23-A	**extra-articular fracture**
23-A1	ulna fractured, radius intact
23-A2	radius, simple and impacted
23-A3	radius, multifragmentary

23-B	**partial articular fracture of radius**
23-B1	sagittal
23-B2	coronal, dorsal rim
23-B3	coronal, palmar rim

23-C	**complete articular fracture of radius**
23-C1	articular simple, metaphyseal simple
23-C2	articular simple, metaphyseal multifragmentary
23-C3	articular multifragmentary

Fig. 1.9c

3. Femur

31. *Proximal* (Fig. 1.10a)

31-A	**extra-articular fracture, trochanteric area**
31-A1	pertrochanteric simple
31-A2	pertrochanteric multifragmentary
31-A3	intertrochanteric

31-B	**extra-articular fracture, neck**
31-B1	subcapital with slight displacement
31-B2	transcervical
31-B3	subcapital, displaced, nonimpacted

31-C	**articular fracture, head**
31-C1	split (Pipkin)
31-C2	with depression
31-C3	with neck fracture

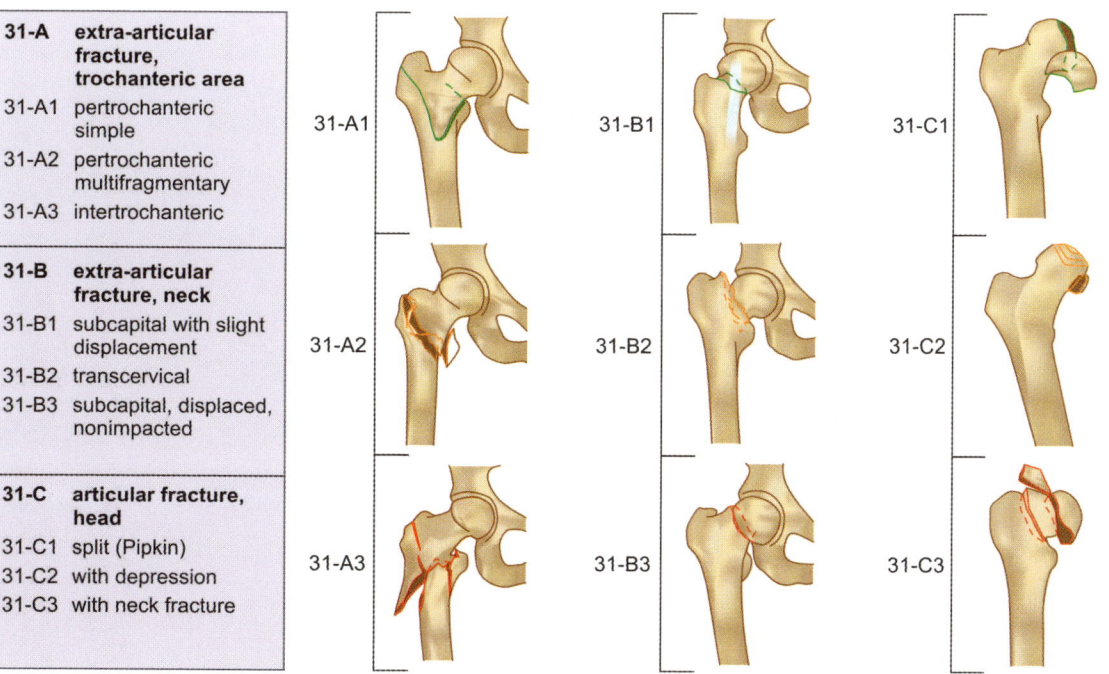

Fig. 1.10a

32. *Diaphyseal* (Fig. 1.10b)

32-A simple fracture	
32-A1 spiral	
32-A2 oblique (≥ 30°)	
32-A3 transverse (< 30°)	
32-A (1-3) 1 subtrochanteric facture	

32-A wedge fracture	
32-A1 spiral wedge	
32-A2 bending wedge	
32-A3 fragmented wedge	
32-A (1-3) 1 subtrochanteric facture	

32-A complex fracture	
32-A1 spiral	
32-A2 segmental	
32-A3 irregular	
32-A (1-3) 1 subtrochanteric facture	

32-A1   32-B1   32-C1

32-A2   32-B2   32-C2

32-A3   32-B3   32-C3

30°

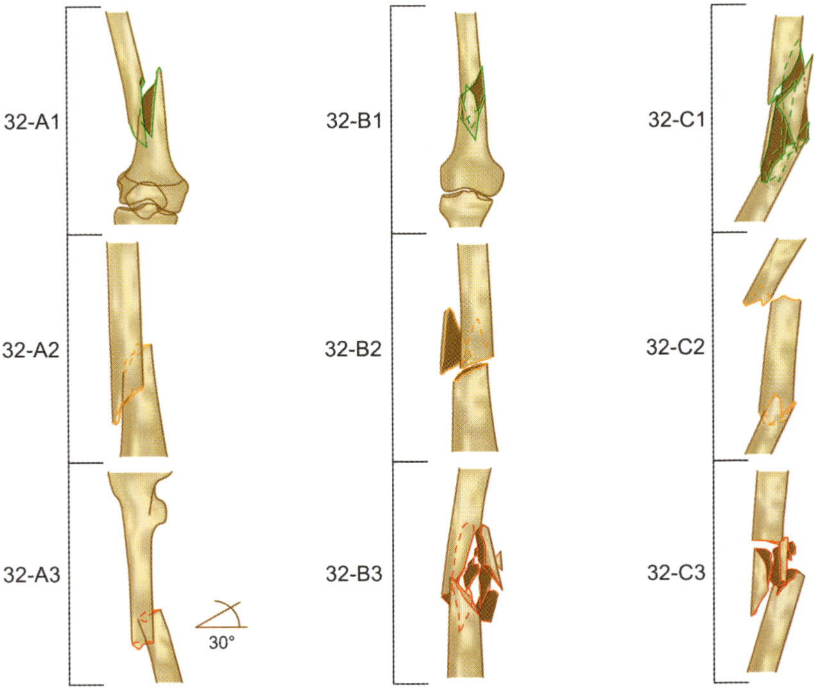

Fig. 1.10b

33. *Distal* (Fig. 1.10c)

33-A extra-articular facture	
33-A1 simple	
33-A2 metaphyseal wedge and/or fragmented wedge	
33-A3 metaphyseal complex	

33-A partial articular facture	
33-A1 lateral	
33-A2 medial condyle, sagittal	
33-A3 coronal	

33-C partial articular facture	
33-C1 articular simple, metaphyseal simple	
33-C2 articular simple, metaphyseal multifragmentary	
33-C3 articular multifragmentary	

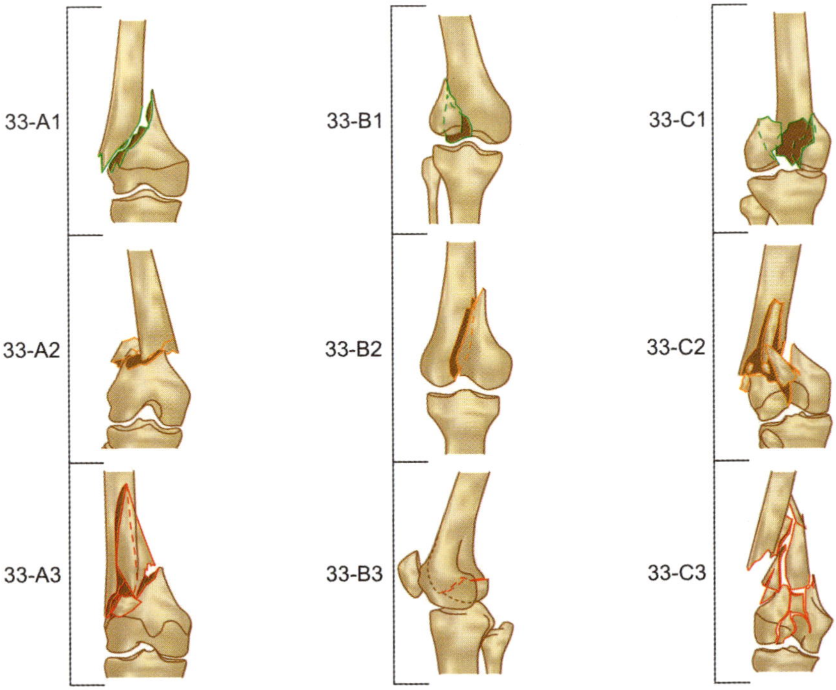

33-A1   33-B1   33-C1

33-A2   33-B2   33-C2

33-A3   33-B3   33-C3

Fig. 1.10c

4. Tibia/Fibula
41. Proximal (Fig. 1.11a)

41-A	extra-articular fracture
41-A1	avulsion
41-A2	metaphyseal simple
41-A3	metaphyseal multifragmentary

41-B	extra-articular fracture
41-B1	pure split
41-B2	pure depression
41-B3	split-depression

41-C	complete articular fracture
41-B1	articular simple, metaphyseal simple
41-B2	articular simple, metaphyseal multifragmentary
41-B3	articular multifragmentary

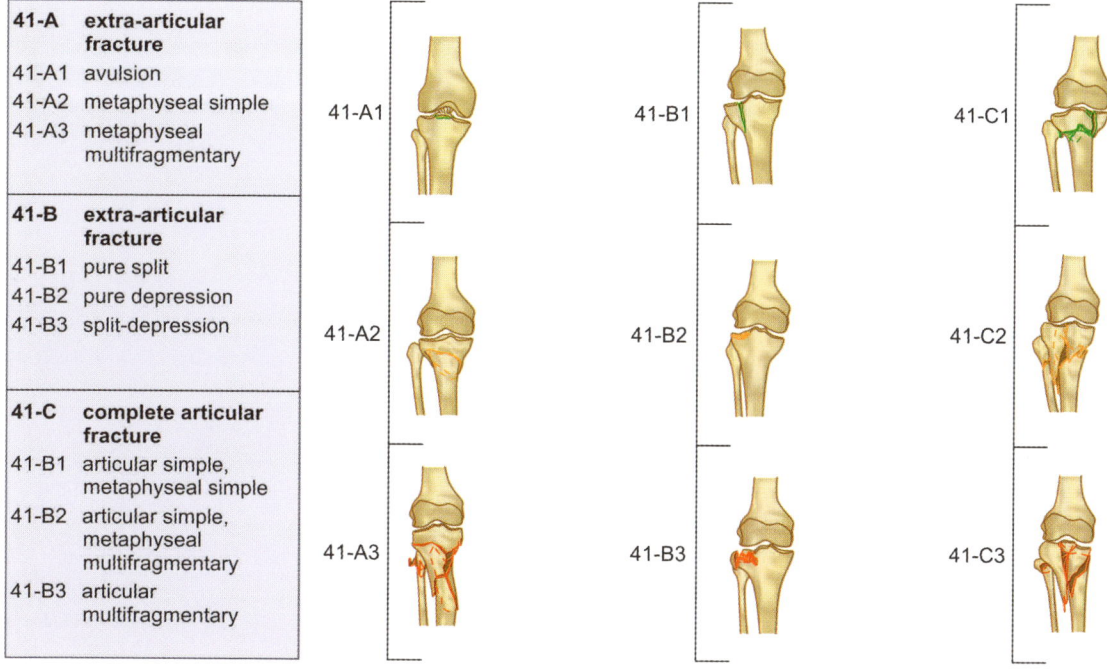

Fig. 1.11a

42. Diaphyseal (Fig. 1.11b)

42-A	simple fracture
42-A1	spiral
42-A2	oblique (≥30°)
42-A3	transverse (<30°)

42-B	wedge fracture
42-B1	spiral wedge
42-B2	bending wedge
42-B3	fragmented wedge

42-C	complex fracture
42-C1	spiral
42-C2	segmental
42-C3	irregular

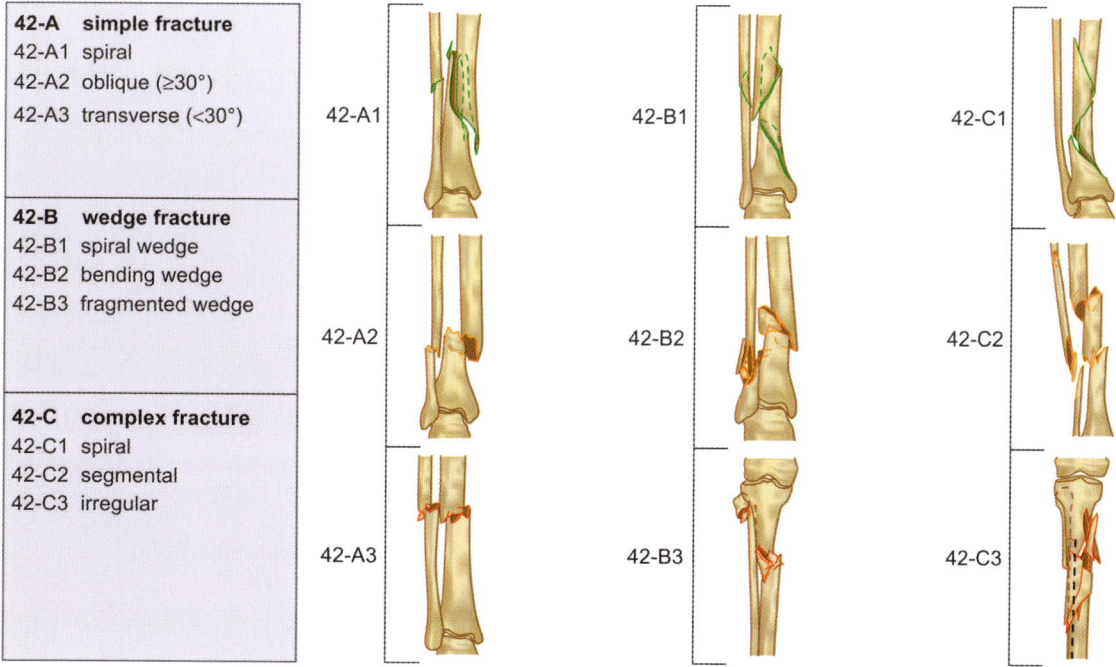

Fig. 1.11b

43. *Distal* (Fig. 1.11c)

43-A	**extra-articular fracture**
43-A1	simple
43-A2	wedge
43-A3	complex

43-B	**partial articular fracture**
43-B1	pure split
43-B2	split-depression
43-B3	multifragmentary depression

43-C	**complete articular fracture**
43-C1	articular simple, metaphyseal simple
43-C2	articular simple, metaphyseal multifragmentary
43-C3	articular multifragmentary

Fig. 1.11c

44. *Malleolar* (Fig. 1.11d)

44-A	**infrasyndesmotic lesion**
44-A1	isolated
44-A2	with fractured medial malleolus
44-A3	with posteromedial fracture

44-A	**transsyndesmotic fibular fracture**
44-B1	isolated
44-B2	with medial lesion
44-B3	with medial lesion and Volkmann's fracture

44-C	**suprasyndesmotic lesion**
44-C1	fibular diaphyseal fracture, simple
44-C2	fibular diaphyseal fracture, multifragmentary
44-C3	proximal fibular lesion

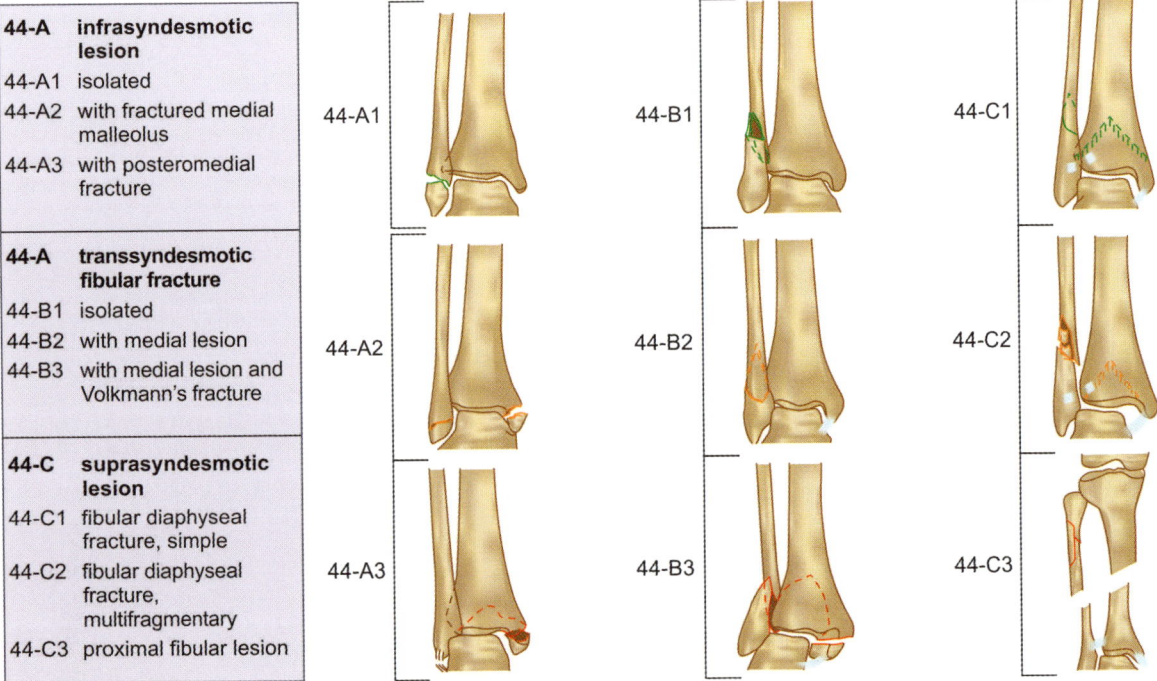

Fig. 1.11d

CLAVICLE

Clavicle is designated number 5 and is divided into standard medial metaphyseal (15-A), diaphyseal (15-B) and lateral metaphyseal (15-C) fractures. An important difference is that the metaphyseal fratures is not 1/3rd of the length of the bone but are shorter fragments according to AO rule of squares (Fig. 1.12).

15-A

- Extra-articular—15-A1
- Intra-articular—15-A2
- Comminuted—14-A3

15-B

- Simple—15-B1
- Wedge—15-B2
- Complex—15-B3

15-C

- Extra-articular—15-C1
- Intra-articular—15-C2.

SHOULDER DISLOCATION

AO/OTA system. The shoulder region is "10". The first digit 1 signifies the shoulder girdle and second digit "0" signifies dislocation. A letter is used to identify the specific joint:

A – Glenohumeral
B – Sternoclavicular
C – Acromioclavicular
D – Scapulothoracic

Followed by another number to describe the direction:

1 – Anterior
2 – Posterior
3 – Lateral (theoretical)
4 – Medial (theoretical)
5 – Other (inferior luxatio erecta)

DISTAL END RADIUS FRACTURE

Modified AO Classification

- *Type A.* Extra-articular fracture. Subgroups are based upon angulation and comminution.

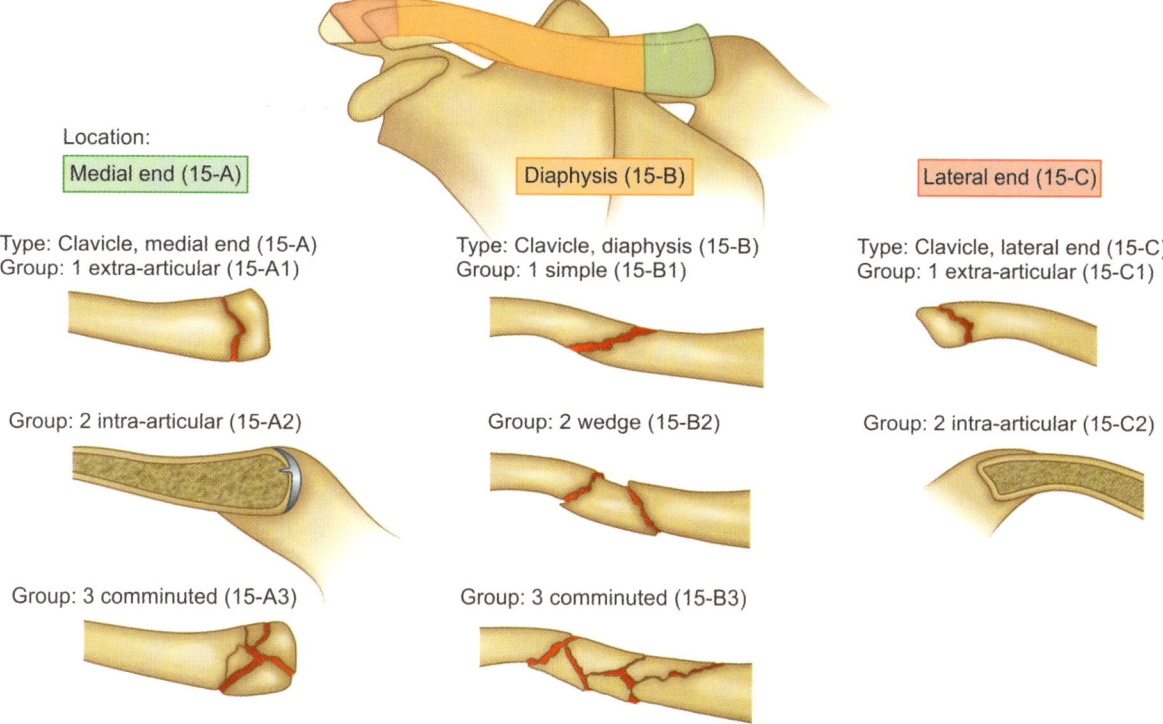

Fig. 1.12: AO/OTA classification of clavicle fractures

- *Type B.* Partial articular fracture

  B1. Radial styloid fracture

  B2. Dorsal rim fracture

  B3. Volar rim fracture

  B4. Die punch fracture.

- *Type C.* Complete articular. Subgroups are based on the articular surface's degree of comminution and the metaphysis.

SUPRACONDYLAR FRACTURE OF HUMERUS

With regard to the degree of displacement at four levels.

- *Type I.* No displacement.
- *Type II.* Displacement in one plane.
- *Type III.* Rotation of the distal fragment with displacement in two planes.
- *Type IV.* Rotation with displacement in three planes, i.e. no contact between bone fragments.

AO COMPREHENSIVE CLASSIFICATION OF ACETABULAR FRACTURES (Table 1.9)

TABLE 1.9

Type A: Partial particular fractures, one column involved
- *A1:* Posterior wall fracture
- *A2:* Posterior column fracture
- *A3:* Anterior wall or anterior column fracture

Type B: Partially articular fractures
- *B1:* Transverse fracture
- *B2:* T-type fracture
- *B3:* Anterior column plus posterior hemi-transverse fracture

Type C: Complete articular fracture (both column fracture; floating acetabulum)
- *C1:* Both column fracture, high variety
- *C2:* Both column fracture, low variety
- *C3:* Both column fracture involving sacroiliac joint

INTERTROCHANTERIC FRACTURES (Fig. 1.13)

Bone = femur = 3, Segment = proximal = 1, Type = trochanteric = A

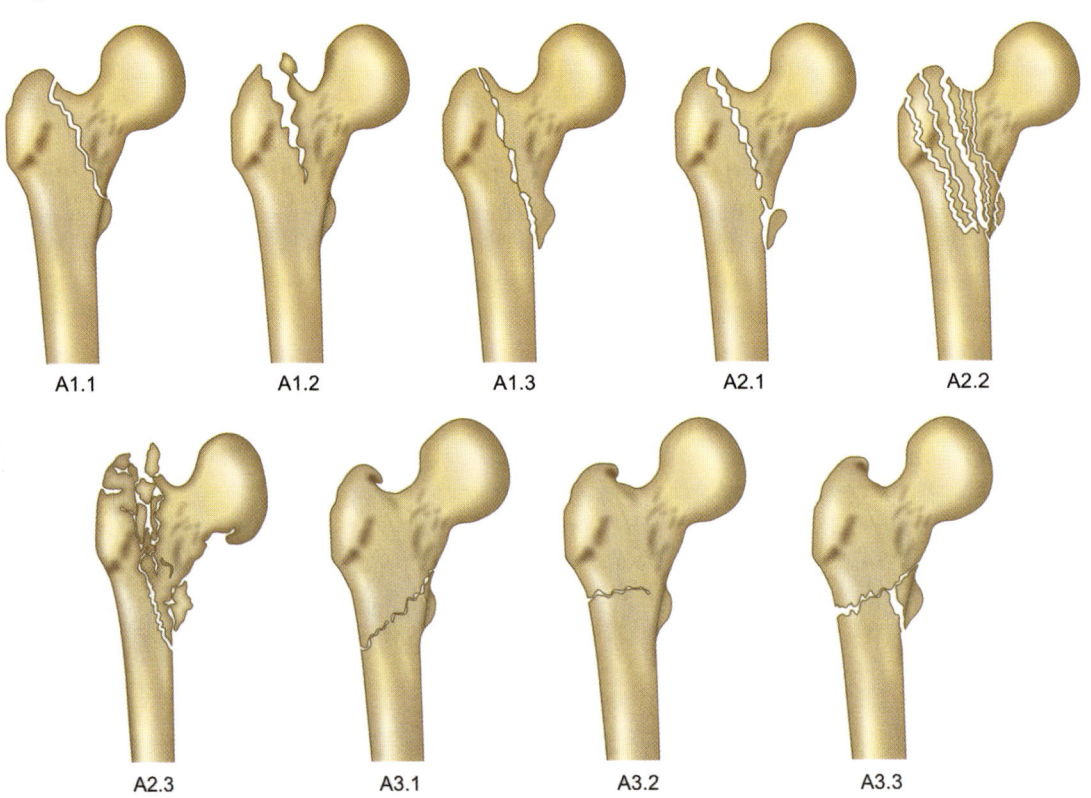

A1.1   A1.2   A1.3   A2.1   A2.2

A2.3   A3.1   A3.2   A3.3

Fig. 1.13: AO/OTA inter-trochanteric fracture classification

A1. Simple (two-part) fractures, with the typical oblique fracture line extending from the greater trochanter to the medial cortex; the lateral cortex of the greater trochanter remains intact.

A2. Fractures are comminuted with a postero-medial fragment; the lateral cortex of the greater trochanter, however, remains intact. Fractures in this group are generally unstable, depending on the size of the medial fragment

A3. Fractures are those in which the fracture line extends across both the medial and lateral cortices; this group includes the reverse obliquity pattern or subtrochanteric extensions (Fig. 1.13).

31-A1 Peritrochanteric simple

31-A1.1 Along intertrochanteric line

31-A1.2 Through greater trochanter

31-A1.3 Below lesser trochanter

31-A2 Peritrochanteric multifragmentary

31-A2.1 With one intermediate fragment

31-A2.2 With several intermediate fragments

31-A2.3 Extending more than 1 cm below lesser trochanter

31-A3 Intertrochanteric

31-A3.1 Simple oblique

31-A3.2 Simple transverse

31-A3.3 Multifragmentary.

Chapter 2

Open and Closed Fractures

A. CLOSED FRACTURES

Tscherne and Gotzen Classification

In Tscherne's classification, soft-tissue injuries are grouped according to severity into four different categories. Along with this, the fracture is labelled as open or closed by an "O" or a "C".

Grade C0. No/minimal soft tissue damage, indirect violence, simple fracture pattern.

Grade CI. Superficial abrasion and contusion caused by pressure from within, mild to moderate fracture pattern.

Grade CII. Deep contaminated abrasion associated with localized skin or muscle contusion through an adequate direct trauma, impending compartment syndrome, severe fracture.

Grade CIII. Extensive skin contusion and crush, subcutaneous tissue avulsion, underlying severed muscle, decompensated compartment syndrome, associated vascular injury, severe fracture.

B. OPEN FRACTURE

1. Gustilo-Anderson Classification

The score should be applied post debridement and the score may change with each debridement.

Type I

- Wound less than 1 cm long
- Moderately clean puncture, where spike of bone has pierced the skin
- Little soft tissue damage
- No crushing
- Fracture usually simple transverse or oblique with little comminution.

Type II

- Laceration more than 1 cm long
- No extensive soft tissue damage, flap or contusion
- Slight to moderate crushing injury
- Moderate comminution
- Moderate contamination

Type III

- Extensive damage to soft tissues
- High degree of contamination
- Fracture caused by high velocity trauma

IIIA. Adequate soft tissue cover
- >10 cm, high energy
- Adequate tissue for coverage
- Includes segmental or extensively comminuted fractures or bone loss even if wound <10 cm
- Gunshot wound

IIIB. Inadequate soft tissue cover, periosteal stripping and bone exposure, massive contamination. A local or free flap is required

IIIC. Any fracture with an arterial injury which requires repair.

2. Tscherne Classification for Tibia

Open fracture grade I (Fr. O I): Fractures of this group are represented by skin lacerated by a bone fragment from the inside. There is no or only little contusion of the skin, and thus fractures are the result of indirect trauma (type A fractures according to the AO/OTA fracture and dislocation classification). However, cases with a minor skin wound, or even with no visible soft-tissue damage, but with a fracture resulting from direct trauma, as type B and type C fractures in the AO/OTA fracture and dislocation classification, must be classified as grade II open.

Open fracture grade II (Fr. O II): Grade II open fractures are characterized by any type of skin laceration with a circumferential skin or soft tissue contusion and moderate contamination. This injury can be accompanied by any type of fracture. Any severe soft-tissue damage without injury to a major vessel or peripheral nerve is categorized in this group.

Open fracture grade III (Fr. O III): To classify a fracture as grade III the fracture must have an extensive soft-tissue damage, often with an additional major vessel injury and/or nerve injury. Every open fracture that is accompanied by ischemia and severe bone comminution belongs in this group. Furthermore, farming accidents, high-velocity gunshot wounds, and manifest compartment syndromes are graded as third degree open because of their extremely high risk of infection.

Open fracture grade IV (Fr. O IV): Grade IV open fractures represent the subtotal and total amputations. Subtotal amputations are defined by the "Replantation Committee of the International Society for Reconstructive Surgery" as separation of all important anatomical structures, especially the major vessels with total ischemia. The remaining soft-tissue bridge may not exceed 1/4 of the circumference of the limb. Any case of revascularization can only be classified as grade three open.

3. Ganga Score

Type IIIB injury involves injury to the covering tissues (skin and fascia), functional tissues (muscle, tendon and nerves) and skeleton (bones and joints) of the limb. A true prognosticating score must evaluate each component of the limb separately and also collectively, whereas Gustilo classification is mainly based on size and nature of the wound.

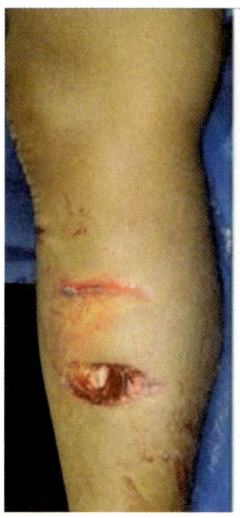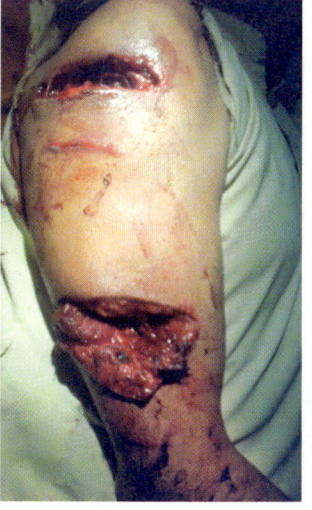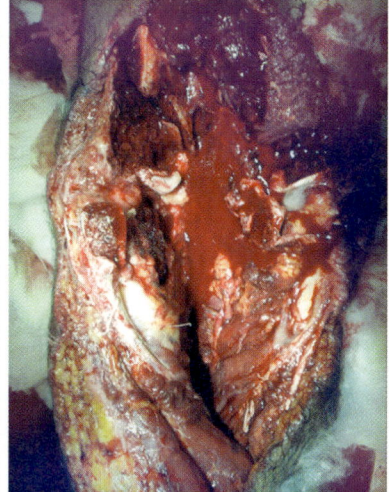

Fig. 2.1: Clinical photograph of different injuries, which are all Gustilo IIIB by definition. Management and outcome of all these injuries, although grouped together under IIIB, are completely different.

Ganga hospital open injury severity score (GHS) gives importance to each component separately, then collectively and the associated factors that influence the treatment and

TABLE 2.1: Ganga score

	Score
Covering structures: skin and fascia	
Wounds not over the bone	
No skin loss	1
With skin loss	2
Wounds over the bone	
No skin loss	3
With skin loss/ friction burns/ degloving over the bone	4
Circumferential wound with bone circumferentially exposed	5
Skeletal structures: bone and joints	
Transverse/oblique fracture with periosteal stripping	1
Butterfly fragment/unicortical comminution (>50% circumference), segmental fractures without bone loss	2
Periarticular comminution with joint disorganization	3
Circumferential comminution/bone loss <4 cm	4
Comminuted/segmental fracture with bone loss >4 cm	5
Functional tissues: musculotendinous (MT) and nerve units	
Exposed musculotendinous (MT) units without injury	1
Repairable injury to MT units	2
Irreparable injury to MT units/ repairable nerve injuries	3
Loss of one compartment of MT units/ irreparable nerve injuries	4
Loss of two or more compartments/subtotal amputation	5

Co-morbid conditions: add two points for each condition present
1. Injury-débridement interval >12 h
2. Sewage or organic contamination/farmyard injuries
3. Age >65 years
4. Debilitating diseases (e.g. drug dependent diabetes mellitus/cardio respiratory diseases leading to increased anesthetic risk)
5. Fat embolism
6. Associated systemic injuries
7. Another major injury to the same limb/compartment syndrome

outcome are also given adequate importance. The score is applied post debridement as it can enable the surgeon to take decision what kind of soft tissue reconstruction is needed and the score can change with each debridement.

- An injured limb, which gets a score of more than three, in two or more components, would be a challenge in salvage and functional outcome might be compromised.
- An injury with a score of 5 in more than one component are having high chances of amputation.
- Patients with score five in MT group, are having high chances of amputation.
- When covering tissue score is more than three, involvement of plastic surgery team is important.
- The total score gives a good indication of the outcome measures analysed:
  Group I. Score of 5 or less.
  Group II. Score between 6 and 10.
  Group III. Score of 11–15.
  Group IV. Score of more than 15.
  All patients in Group IV are having grave injury and can eventually lead to amputation.

4. AO Classification of Open Fractures

AO group uses separate classification for closed/open skin injuries and for injuries involving muscles. They use a separate fourth classification for neurovascular involvement. It is a complex scoring system and is not used in daily clinical practice.

Skin lesions in closed fractures (integument closed-IC, Fig. 2.2)
- *IC1.* Skin undamaged
- *IC2.* Contusion of skin
- *IC3.* Local degloving
- *IC4.* Extensive (but closed) degloving
- *IC5.* Skin necrosis resulting for contusion.

Skin lesions in open fractures (integument open – IO, Fig. 2.3)
- *IO1.* Skin open from within out
- *IO2.* Skin broken from without in, with contused edges but less than 5 cm in length

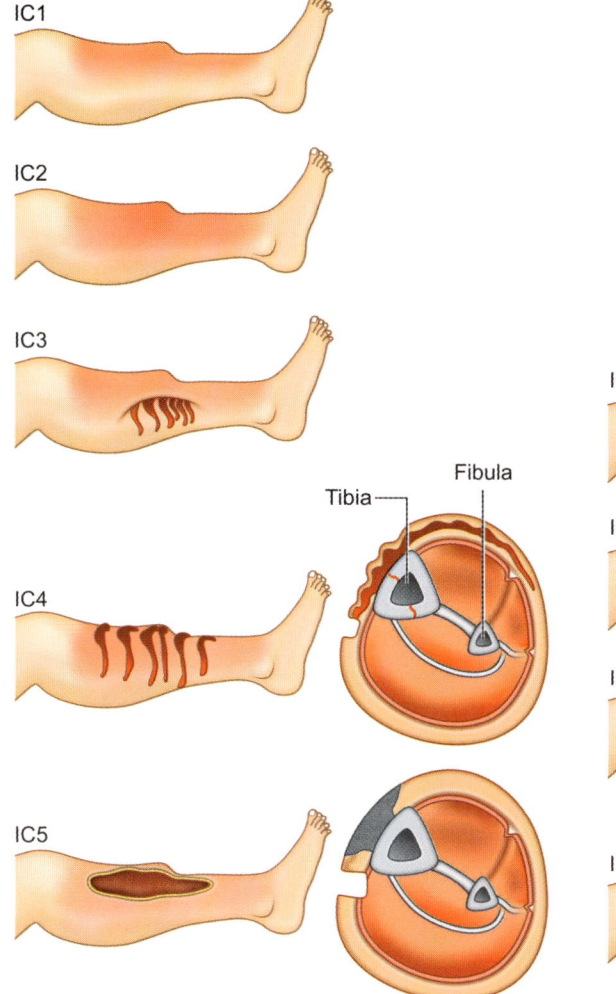

IC1

IC2

IC3

Tibia   Fibula

IC4

IC5

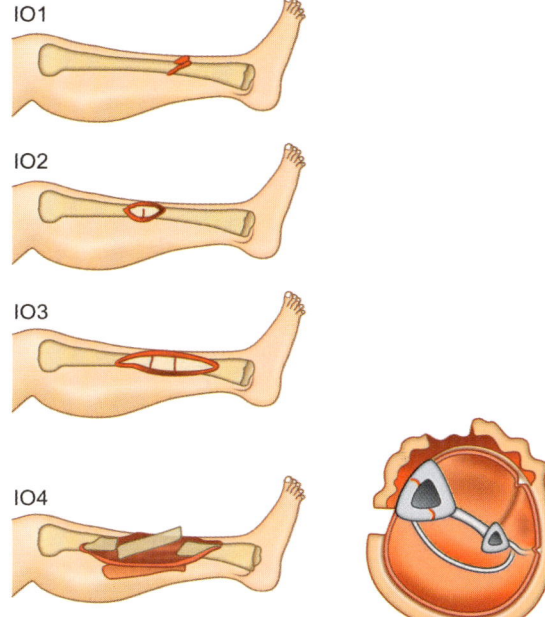

IO1

IO2

IO3

IO4

Fig. 2.2: Pictorial representation of integumentary closed fractures in increasing severity.

Fig. 2.3: Pictorial representation of integumentary open fractures in increasing severity.

- *IO3*. In excess of 5 cm of skin broken, with devitalised edges and local degloving
- *IO4*. Full thickness contusion, abrasion, skin loss
- *IO5*. Extensive degloving.

Muscle and tendon injuries in fractures (Fig. 2.4)
- *MT1*. No muscle injury
- *MT2*. Local muscle injury, one muscle group only
- *MT3*. Extensive muscle injury with involvement of more than one group
- *MT4*. Avulsion or loss of entire muscle groups, tendon laceration

- *MT5*. Compartment syndrome, Crush syndrome.

Neurovascular injuries in fractures (Fig. 2.4)
- *NV1*. No neurovascular injury
- *NV2*. Isolated nerve injury
- *NV3*. Isolated vascular injury
- *NV4*. Extensive segmental vascular injury
- *NV5*. Combined neurovascular injury including subtotal or total amputation.
  Gustilo type I equivalent to IO1.
  Gustilo type II equivalent to IO2.
  Gustilo type IIIA equivalent to IO3.
  Gustilo type IIIB equivalent to IO4.
  Gustilo type IIIC equivalent to IO3–5 + NV3.

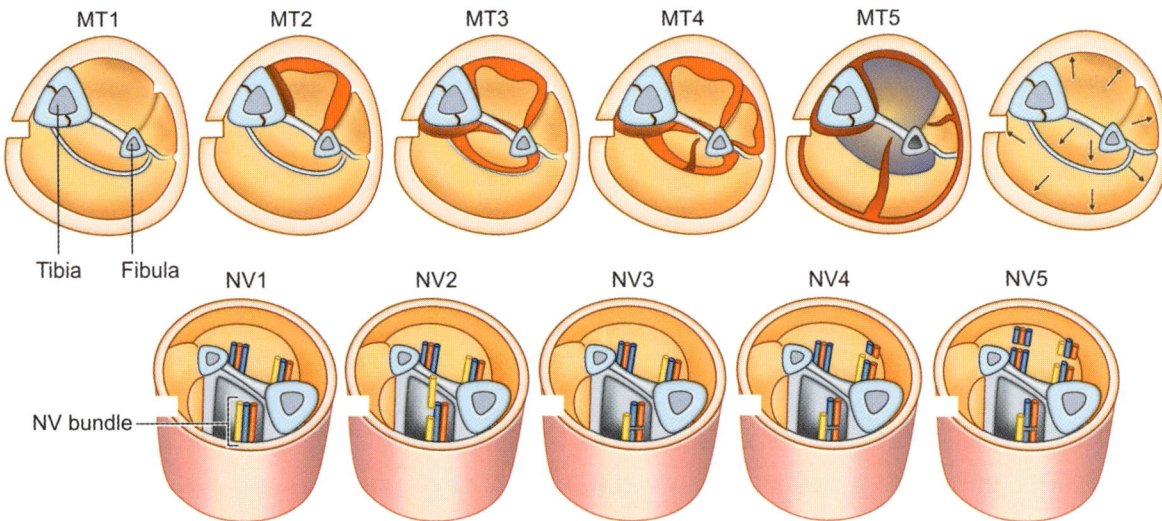

Fig. 2.4: Pictorial representation of musculotendinous injury and neurovascular injury associated with fractures in increasing severity.

5. Mangled Extrimity Severity Score

Table 2.2 shows Mangled extremity severity score.

Amputation is the likely result if score is more than or equal to 7

Type	Characteristics	Lesions	Sutures
TABLE 2.2: Mangled extremity severity score			
Group of skeletal lesion and soft tissue			
1	Low energy	Sharp wound, simple closed fracture, projectile low-caliber firearm	1
2	Medium energy	Multiple or exposed fractures, dislocation, moderate crush injury	2
3	High energy	Explosion gunshot wound from a high-speed firearm	3
4	Massive crushing	Fall from a tree, train accident, smothering	4
Shock group			
1	Hemodynamically normotensive	Stable blood pressure	0
2	Transient hypotension	Unstable pressure, but responding to intravenous fluid	1
3	Prolonged hypotension	Systolic pressure of <90 mmHg and responding to intravenous infusion of fluid only in the operating room	
Ischemic group			
1*	Absence	Pulse without signs of ischemia	0*
2*	Mild	Pulse reduced without signs of ischemia	1*
3*	Moderately	No pulse on Doppler imaging prolonged capillary refill, paresthesia, decreased motor activity	2*
4*	Serious	Pulseless, cold limb, which is paralyzed and numb without capillary refill	3*
Age group			
1		<30 years	0
2		30–50 years	1
3		>50 years	2

*Multiply by 2 if ischemia persists of >6 hours
Limbs with scores of 7–12 points usually require amputation. Limbs with scores f 3–6 points are usually salvagable.

Chapter 3

Shoulder and Upper Limb

1. Clavicle

Clavicle is mainly divided into three parts medial, middle and lateral 1/3rd, and clavicle fractures are divided on the basis of their anatomical location.

A. Allman/Craig divided fracture into three types

   Group I—middle 1/3rd

   Group II—lateral/3rd

   Group III—medial 1/3rd.

B. Neer classified lateral 1/3rd fractures into three types and Rockwood further sub-divided Neer's type II into two subtypes.

A. Allman/Craig Classification

Group I. Middle Third Fractures (80%)

- Undisplaced
- Displaced

Group II. Distal Third Fractures (15%)

They are sub-divided according to the location of coracoclavicular ligaments and acromioclavicular ligaments.

- **Type I.** Minimally displaced/interligamentous, i.e. the fracture line is between clavicular attachment of coracoclavicular ligament and acromioclavicular ligament. Coracoclavicular ligaments are intact and attached to the medial segment.

- **Type II.** Displaced fractures, fracture medial to the coracoclavicular ligaments and thus higher incidence of non-union.

    IIA. Both ligaments (conoid and trapezoid) attached to the distal fragment

    IIB. Conoid torn, trapezoid attached to the distal fragment (fracture line is lateral to both coracoclavicular ligaments and both the ligaments are torned).

- **Type III.** Fractures involving AC joint articular surface with no ligamentous injury and thus it may be confused with AC joint injury.

- **Type IV.** A physeal fracture that occurs in skeletally immature group. Intact coracoclavicular ligaments attached to periosteal sleeve plus proximal fragment displaced through tear in thick periosteum.

- **Type V.** Comminuted fracture and ligaments remain attached to the comminuted fragment.

Group III. Fracture of the Proximal Third (5%)

- Type I. Minimally displacement
- Type II. Displaced
- Type III. Intra-articular
- Type IV. Epiphyseal separation
- Type V. Comminuted

    Anterior displacement in Group III is mainly asymptomatic whereas posterior displacement are rare occurrence, often physeal fracture dislocation and may compromise airway or neurovascular structures.

B. Neer's Lateral 1/3rd Clavicle Fracture Classification (Fig. 3.1)

- *Type I.* Minimally displaced/interligamentous, i.e. the fracture line is between clavicular attachment of coracoclavicular ligament and acromioclavicular ligament. Coracoclavicular ligaments are intact and attached to the medial segment.
- *Type II.* Displaced fractures, fracture medial to the coracoclavicular ligaments and thus higher incidence of non-union.
  IIA. Both ligaments (conoid and trapezoid) attached to the distal fragment.
  IIB. Conoid torn, trapezoid attached to the distal fragment (fracture line is lateral to both coracoclavicular ligaments and both the ligaments are torned).
- *Type III.* Fractures involving AC joint articular surface with no ligamentous injury and thus it may be confused with AC joint injury.

C. Robinson Fracture Classification

Robinson classification uses uses fracture type numbering according to medial—lateral location contrary to the traditional system described above and is of prognostic value especially in middle 1/3rd fracture.

- *Type 1.* Medial 1/5th clavicle fractures
  a. Undisplaced
    a1. Extra-articular
    a2. Intra-articular
  b. Displaced
    b1. Extra-articular
    b2. Intra-articular
- *Type 2.* Middle 3/5th clavicle fractures
  a. Cortical alignment fractures
    a1. Undisplaced
    a2. Angulated
  b. Displaced fractures
    b1. Simple, wedge comminution
    b2. Multifragmentary, segmental
- *Type 3.* Lateral 1/5th clavicle fractures
  a. Undisplaced
    a1. Extra-articular
    a2. Intra-articular
  b. Displaced
    b1. Extra-articular
    b2. Intra-articular

D. AO/OTA Classification

Clavicle is designated number 5 and is divided into standard medial metaphyseal (15-A), diaphyseal (15-B) and lateral metaphyseal (15-C) fractures. An important difference is that the metaphyseal fratures is not 1/3rd of the length of the bone but are shorter fragments according to AO rule of squares.

- 15-A
  - Extra-articular—15-A1
  - Intra-articular—15-A2
  - Comminuted—14-A3
- 15-B
  - Simple—15-B1
  - Wedge—15-B2
  - Complex—15-B3
- 15-C
  - Extra-articular—15-C1
  - Intra-articular—15-C2.

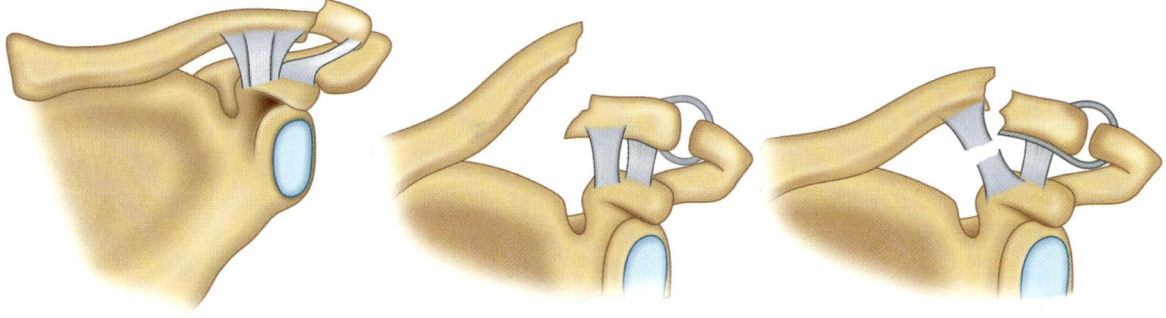

Neer Type I Neer Type IIA Neer Type IIB

Fig. 3.1: Neer's classification of lateral 1/3rd clavicle fracture.

2. ACROMIAL FRACTURE

Kuhn et al Classification (Fig. 3.2)

Type I. Type I fractures are minimally displaced.

- Type IA fractures are avulsion fractures and heal rapidly.
- Type IB fractures result from direct trauma to the extremity, and are minimally displaced. Most heal with nonoperative treatment.

Type II. Type II fractures are displaced laterally, superiorly or anteriorly and do not reduce the subacromial space.

Type III. Type III fractures reduce the sub-acromial space. This may occur by an inferiorly displaced acromion fracture, or an acromion fracture associated with an ipsilateral, superiorly displaced glenoid neck fracture.

3. ACROMIOCLAVICULAR JOINT

Rockwood Classification (Fig. 3.3)

Type I
- Sprain of the acromioclavicular (AC) ligament.
- AC joint tenderness, minimal pain with arm motion, no pain in coracoclavicular inter-spaces.
- No abnormality on radiographs.

Type II
- AC ligament tear with joint disruption and sprained coracoclavicular ligaments. Distal clavicle is slightly superior to acromion and mobile to palpation; tenderness is found in the coracoclavicular space.
- Radiographs (B/L AC joint ZANCA view) demonstrate slight elevation of the distal end of the clavicle (<50% clavicle width)

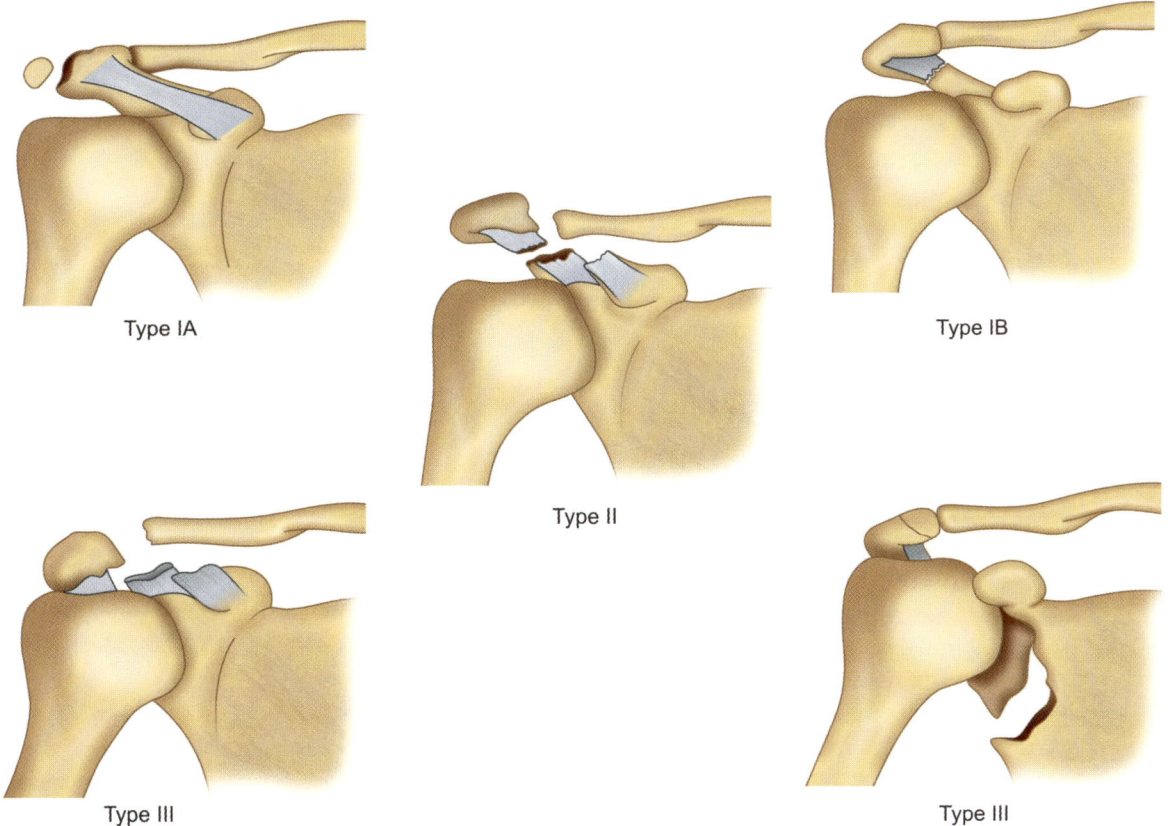

Type IA

Type IB

Type II

Type III

Type III

Fig. 3.2: Kuhn et al classification of acromial fracture.

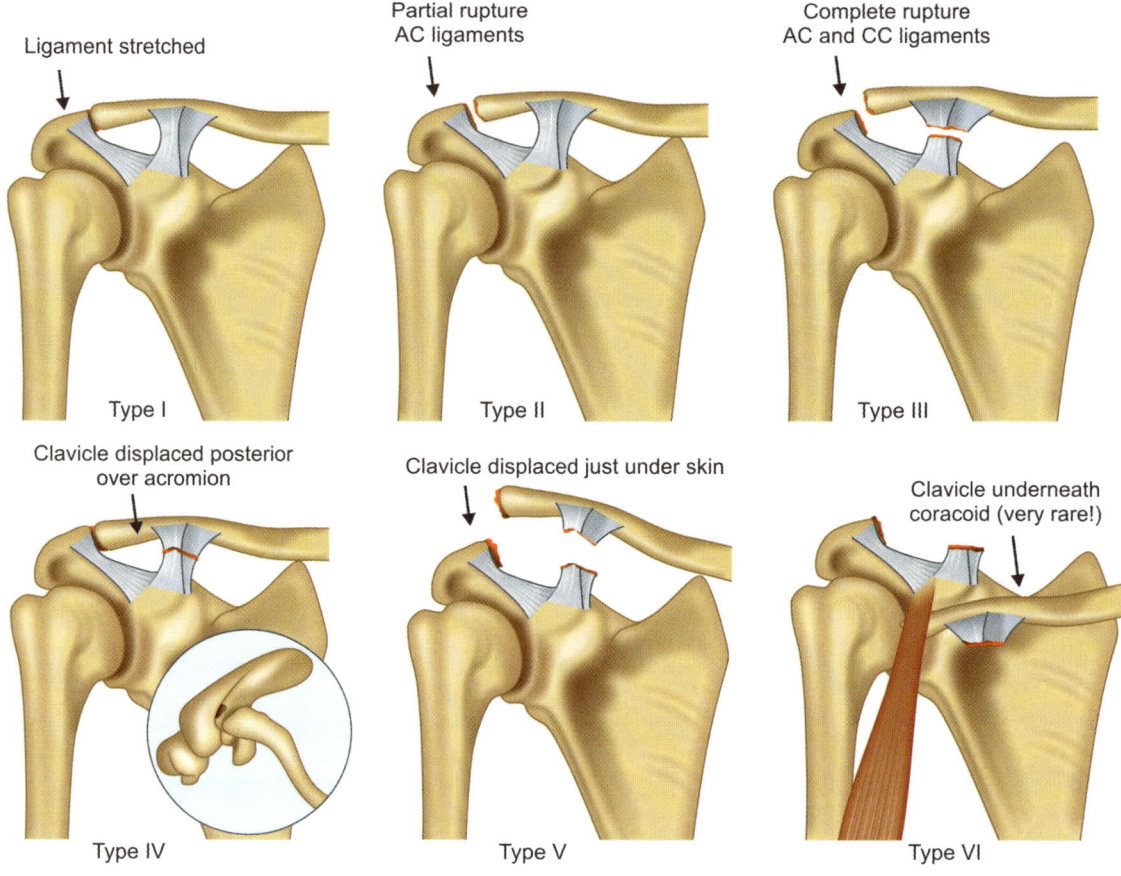

Fig. 3.3: Rockwood classification of acromioclavicular joint injury.

and AC joint widening. Stress films show the coracoclavicular ligaments are sprained but integrity is maintained.

Type III
- AC and coracoclavicular ligaments torn with AC joint dislocation; deltoid and trapezius muscles usually detached from the distal clavicle.
- The upper extremity and distal fragment are depressed, and the distal end of the proximal fragment may tent the skin. The AC joint is tender, coracoclavicular widening is evident.
- Radiographs demonstrate the distal clavicle superior to the medial border of the acromion; stress views reveal a widened coracoclavicular interspace 25 to 100% greater than the normal side.

Type IV
- Type III with the distal clavicle displaced posteriorly into or through the trapezius.
- Clinically, more pain exists than in type III; the distal clavicle is displaced posteriorly away from the clavicle.
- Axillary radiograph or computed tomography demonstrates posterior displacement of the distal clavicle.

Type V
- Type III with the distal clavicle grossly and severely displaced superiorly.
- This type is typically associated with tenting of the skin.
- Radiographs demonstrate the coracoclavicular interspace to be 100 to 300% greater than the normal side.

Type VI
- AC dislocated, with the clavicle displaced inferior to the acromion or the coracoid; the coracoclavicular interspace is decreased compared with normal.
- The deltoid and trapezius muscles are detached from the distal clavicle.
- The mechanism of injury is usually a severe direct force onto the superior surface of the distal clavicle, with abduction of the arm and scapula retraction.
- Clinically, the shoulder has a flat appearance with a prominent acromion; associated clavicle and upper rib fractures and brachial plexus injuries are due to high energy trauma.
- Radiographs demonstrate one of two types of inferior dislocation: Subacromial or subcoracoid.

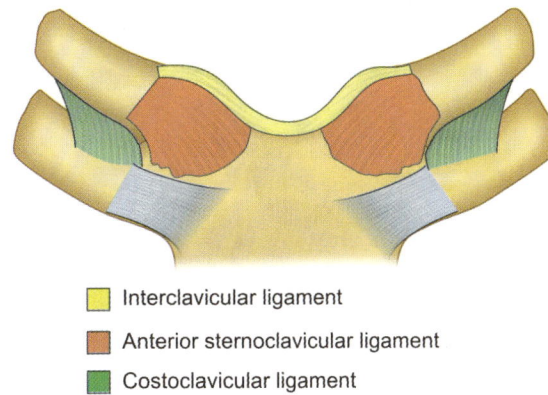

☐ Interclavicular ligament
☐ Anterior sternoclavicular ligament
☐ Costoclavicular ligament

Fig. 3.4: Ligamentous attachment of sternoclavicular region.

4. STERNOCLAVICULAR JOINT

Anatomic Classification

Anterior dislocation—more common.

The medial end of clavicle is displaced anteriorly/anterosuperiorly with respect to anterior margin of sternum.

Posterior dislocation—less common

The medial end of clavicle is displaced posteriorly/posterosuperiorly with respect to anterior margin of sternum.

More dangerous as may be associated with neurovascular complication.

Etiologic Classification

Atraumatic: Spontaneous atraumatic subluxation or dislocation can occur especially in females of late teen or early adult age group who has generalized ligament laxity of other joints.
- Anterior—more common.
- Posterior—rare.

Traumatic: **Allman** classification
- *Mild*: Joint stable/sprain, ligamentous integrity maintained.

- *Moderate*: Subluxation, with partial ligamentous disruption.
- *Severe*: Acute unstable joint/dislocation, with complete ligamentous compromise. Occasionally the costoclavicular ligament is intact but stretched out enough to allow dislocation of the joint (Fig. 3.4).

Chronic dislocation: If the initial acute traumatic dislocation does not heal, mild to moderate forces may produce recurrent dislocations, but that is rare.

5. SCAPULOTHORACIC DISLOCATION (Fig. 3.5)

Damschen et al Classification
- *Type I.* An isolated musculoskeletal injury.
- *Type II.* Involves a musculoskeletal injury with either a vascular injury or a neurological injury.
  - *Type IIA.* Vascular disruption.
  - *Type IIB.* Neurological disruption.
- *Type III.* Injury includes a patient with a musculoskeletal injury and both a vascular and a neurological injury.

It can be diagnosed clinically and radiologically with AP X-ray of chest with BL scapula.

Scapular index: Ratio between the distance of medial border of injured/normal scapula with the spinous process (Fig. 3.5a and b).

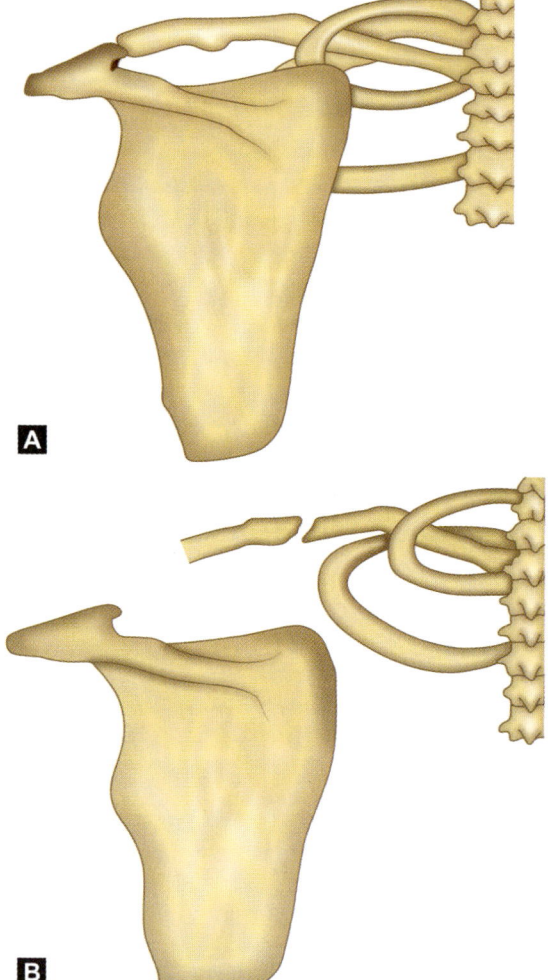

A

B

Fig. 3.5a: Figure (A) is normal scapula, (B) is lateral displacement of scapula.

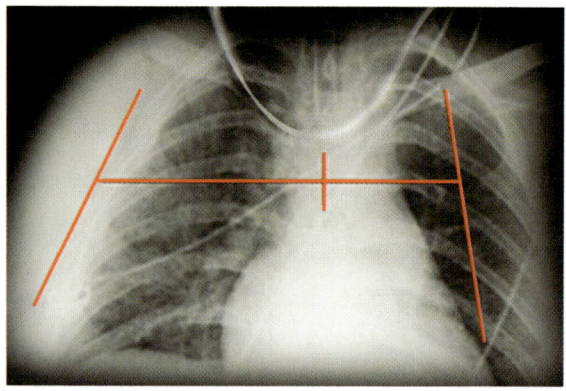

Fig. 3.5b: X-ray showing right side scapulothoracic dislocation with scapular index.

6. SCAPULA

A. Zdravkovic and Damholt Classification
- **Type I.** Scapula body
- **Type II.** Apophyseal fractures, including the acromion and coracoid
- **Type III.** Fractures of the superolateral angle, including the scapular neck and glenoid.

B. Coracoid Fractures: Eyres and Brooks Classification (Fig. 3.6a)
- **Type I.** Coracoid tip or epiphyseal fracture
- **Type II.** Mid process
- **Type III.** Basal fracture
- **Type IV.** Involvement of superior body of scapula
- **Type V.** Extension into the glenoid fossa

The suffix of A or B can be used to record the presence of absence of damage to the clavicle or its ligamentous connection to the scapula.

C. Intra-articular Glenoid Fractures: Ideberg Classification (Fig. 3.6b)
- **Type I.** Avulsion fracture of the anterior margin.
  - *Type IA.* Anterior rim #
  - *Type IB.* Posterior rim #.
- **Type II.** # line through glenoid fossa exiting scapula laterally.
  - *Type IIA.* Transverse fracture through the glenoid fossa exiting inferiorly.
  - *Type IIB.* Oblique fracture through the glenoid fossa exiting inferiorly.
- **Type III.** Oblique fracture through the glenoid exiting superiorly; often associated with an acromioclavicular joint injury.
- **Type IV.** Transverse fracture exiting through the medial border of the scapula.
- **Type V.** Combination of a type II and type IV pattern.
  - VA—II + IV
  - VB— III + IV
  - VC—II, III, IV.
- **Type VI.** Severe continuation of glenoid surface (GOSS).

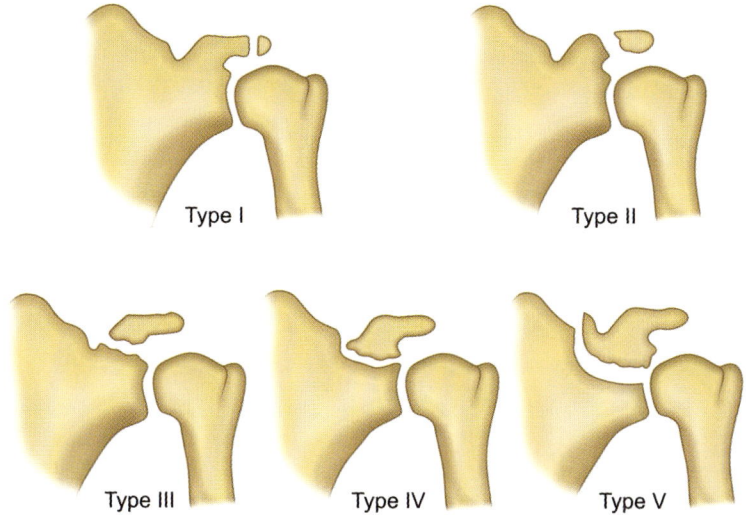

Fig. 3.6a: Eyres and Brooks classification of coracoids process fracture.

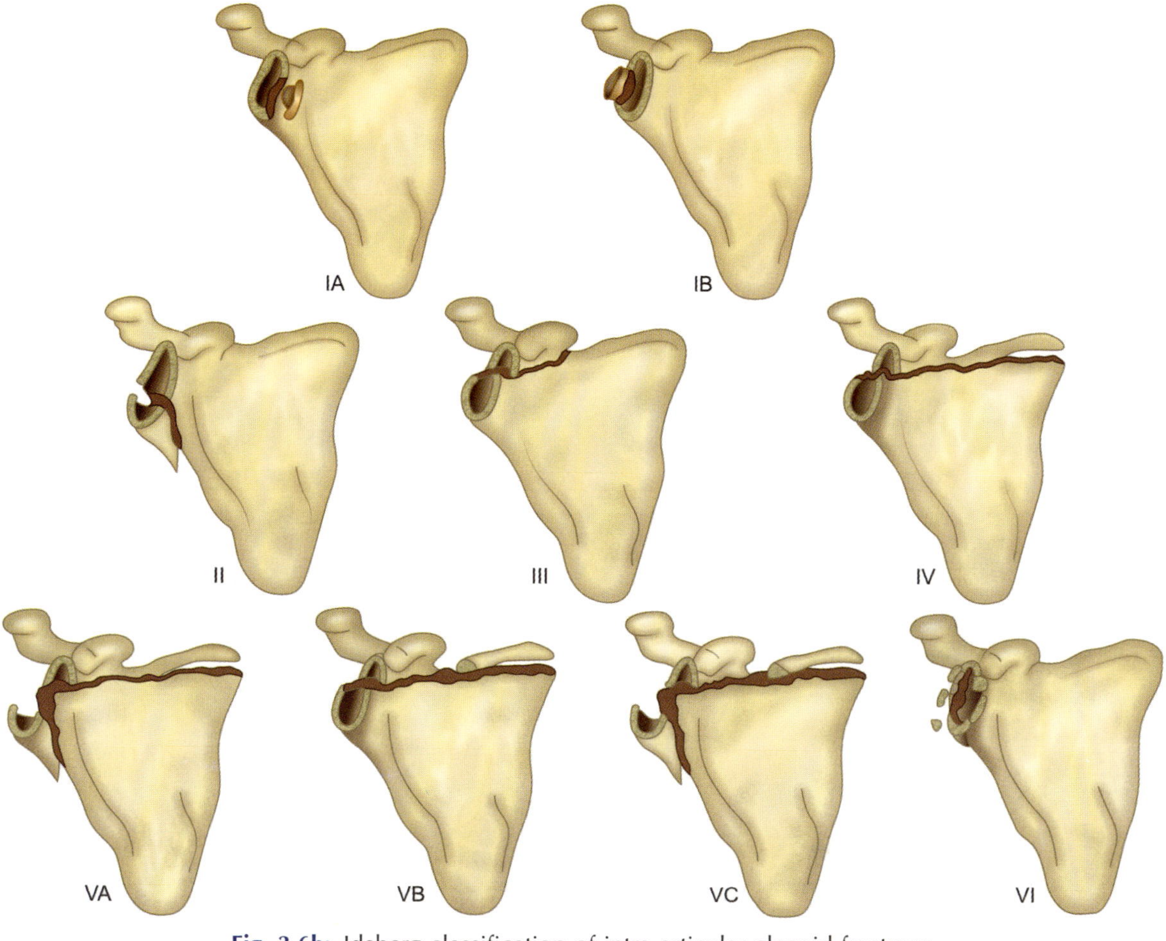

Type I

Type II

Type III

Type IV

Type V

IA

IB

II

III

IV

VA

VB

VC

VI

Fig. 3.6b: Ideberg classification of intra-articular glenoid fractures.

D. Comprehensive Anatomical Classification

This classification is based on classification developed by Tscherne and Christ, Ada and Miller, and Euler and Ruedi. However, the basic groups of this classification includes only the fracture lines whose existence has been verified by 3D CT reconstruction or intraoperatively.

Process fractures
- *A1.* Fracture of the superior border and the superior angle.
- *A2.* Fracture of the acromian and the lateral part of the scapular spine.
- *A3.* Fracture of the coracoids process.

Body fractures
- *B1.* Fractures of the anatomical body
- *B2.* Fractures of the biomechanical body.

Neck fractures
- *C1.* Fracture of the anatomical neck
- *C2.* Fracture of the surgical neck
- *C3.* Transspinous fracture of the scapular neck.

Glenoid fossa fractures
- *D1.* Fractures of the superior glenoid.
- *D2.* Avulsion of the anteroinferior rim of the glenoid.
- *D3.* Fractures of the inferior glenoid.
- *D4.* Fractures of the posterior rim of the glenoid.

7. GLENOHUMERAL INSTABILITY

Classification

- *Degree of instability*: Dislocation/subluxation
- *Chronology/type*
  - Congenital
  - Acute versus chronic
  - Locked (fixed)
  - Recurrent
- *Force/etiological*
  - Atraumatic
  - Traumatic
  - Neuromuscular
  - Microtraumatic
- *Patient contribution*
  - Voluntary
  - Involuntary

- *Direction*
  - Anterior (Fig. 3.7a)
    - Subcoracoid
    - Subglenoid
    - Subclavicular
    - Intrathoracic
  - Posterior (Fig. 3.7b)
    - Subacromial-M/C
    - Subspinous
    - Subglenoid

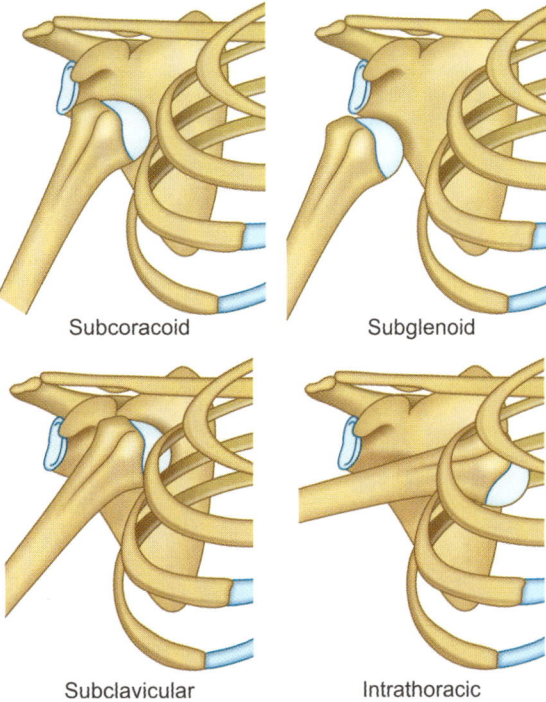

Subcoracoid   Subglenoid

Subclavicular   Intrathoracic

Fig. 3.7a: Different types of anterior shoulder dislocation.

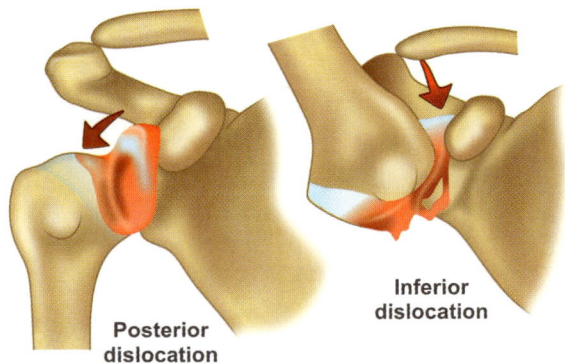

Posterior dislocation

Inferior dislocation

Fig. 3.7b: Posterior and inferior shoulder dislocation.

– Inferior also known as luxatio erecta
– Superior
– Multidirectional instability (MDI).

AO/OTA system: The shoulder region is "10". The first digit 1 signifies the shoulder girdle and second digit "0" signifies dislocation. A letter is used to identify the specific joint:

A. Glenohumeral

B. Sternoclavicular

C. Acromioclavicular

D. Scapulothoracic

Followed by another number to describe the direction:
1. Anterior
2. Posterior
3. Lateral (theoretical)
4. Medial (theoretical)
5. Other (inferior-luxatio erecta).

8. PROXIMAL HUMERUS FRACTURE

Neer Classification (Fig. 3.8)

This classification is useful in guiding treatment.

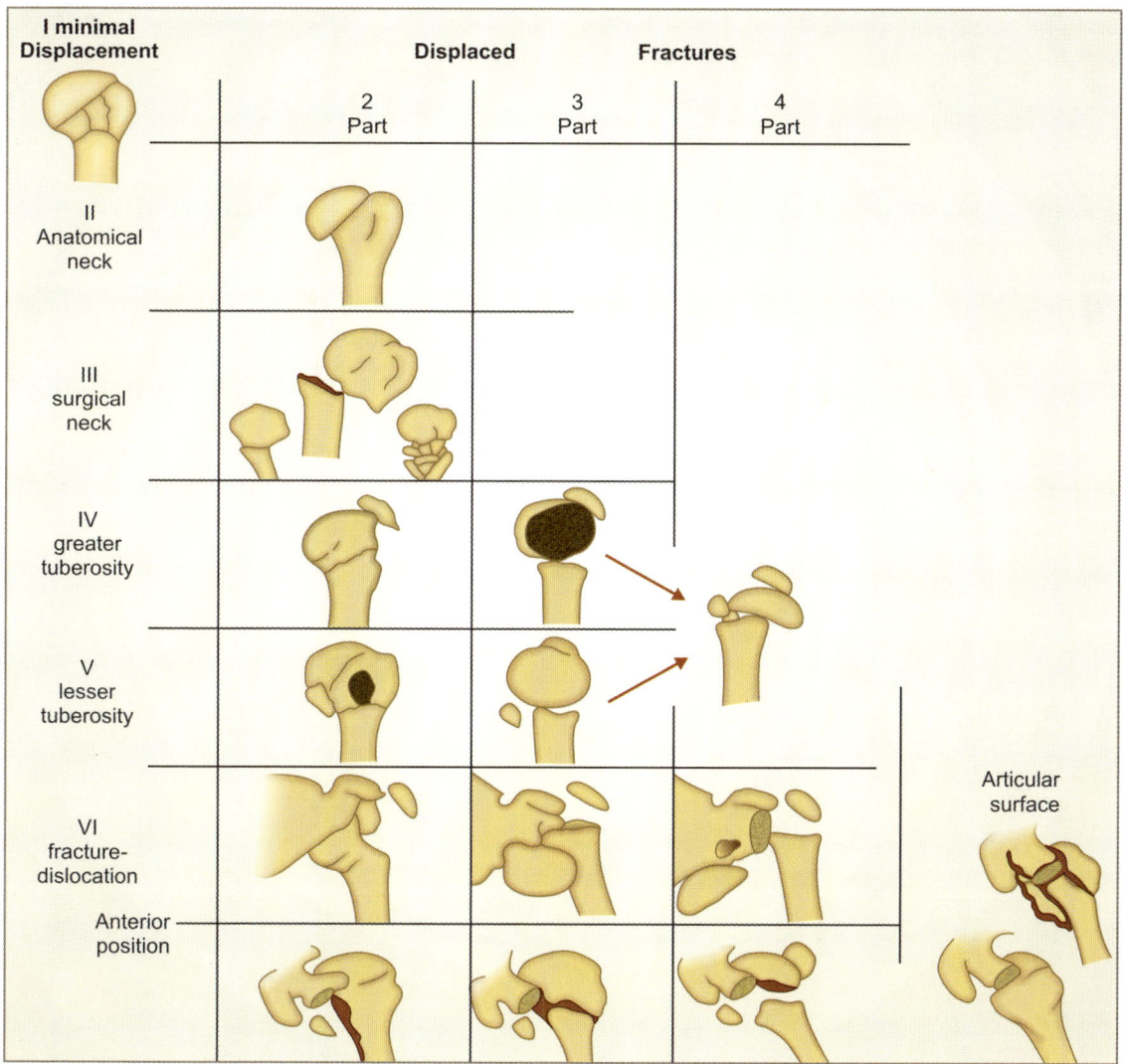

Fig. 3.8: Neer classification of proximal humerus fracture.

The four parts are the greater and lesser tuberosities, the shaft, and the humeral head. A part is displaced if >1 cm of displacement or >45 degree of angulation is seen.

One-part fracture
- Fracture line involves 1 of 4 parts
- None of the parts are displaced

Two-part fracture
- Fracture lines involve 2 of 4 parts and one part is displaced.
- Segment named is the one displaced.
- Fracture line M/C involves the surgical neck.
- GT # is associated with anterior shoulder dislocation and a lower threshold (>5 mm) for displacement has been proposed.

Three-part fracture
- Fracture line involves 3 of 4 parts and 2 parts are displaced.
- Displacement of shaft in all classification based on the type of tuberosity displaced.
  1. GT and shaft displaced with respect to LT and articular surface which remain together (M/C).
  2. LT and shaft displaced with respect to GT and articular surface which remain together.

Four-part fracture
- Fracture line involves all four parts.
- 3 parts are displaced with respect to fourth part.
- Ischaemic osteonecrosis is M/C after displaced four-part fracture.
- Displaced 3–4 part fracture alter articular congruity of glenohumeral joint and has the highest likelihood of disrupting major blood supply of proximal humerus.

9. HUMERAL SHAFT

Descriptive Classification

Open/closed

Location: Proximal third, middle third, distal third

Degree: Incomplete, complete

Direction and character: Transverse, oblique, spiral, segmental, comminuted

Intrinsic condition of the bone

Articular extension

AO Classification of Humeral Diaphyseal Fractures (Fig. 3.9a)

Type A. Simple fracture
- *A1.* Spiral
- *A2.* Oblique (>30°)
- *A3.* Transverse (<30°)

Type B. Wedge fracture
- *B1.* Spiral wedge
- *B2.* Bending wedge
- *B3.* Fragmented wedge

Type C. Complex fracture
- *C1.* Spiral
- *C2.* Segmented
- *C3.* Irregular (significant comminution)

Garnavos Classification (Table 3.1)

It is a classification system supplementing AO/OTA system for any long bone fracture. Thus fracture shaft of humerus is being also classified by this system.

Holstein and Lewis fracture (Fig. 3.9b): A special type of fracture of distal shaft of humerus, a simple displaced spiral fracture, with the distal end deviating towards the radial side with an increased risk of radial nerve palsy.

TABLE 3.1: Garnavos classification

Topograpy	Morphology
P: Proximal	**S: S**imple(no fragments) **t: t**ransverse or oblique **s: s**piral
M: Middle	**I: I**ntermediate (1 or 2 sizable fragments)
D: Distal	**C: C**omplex (>3 any size fragments or large comminution)
j: Extension toward the joint	

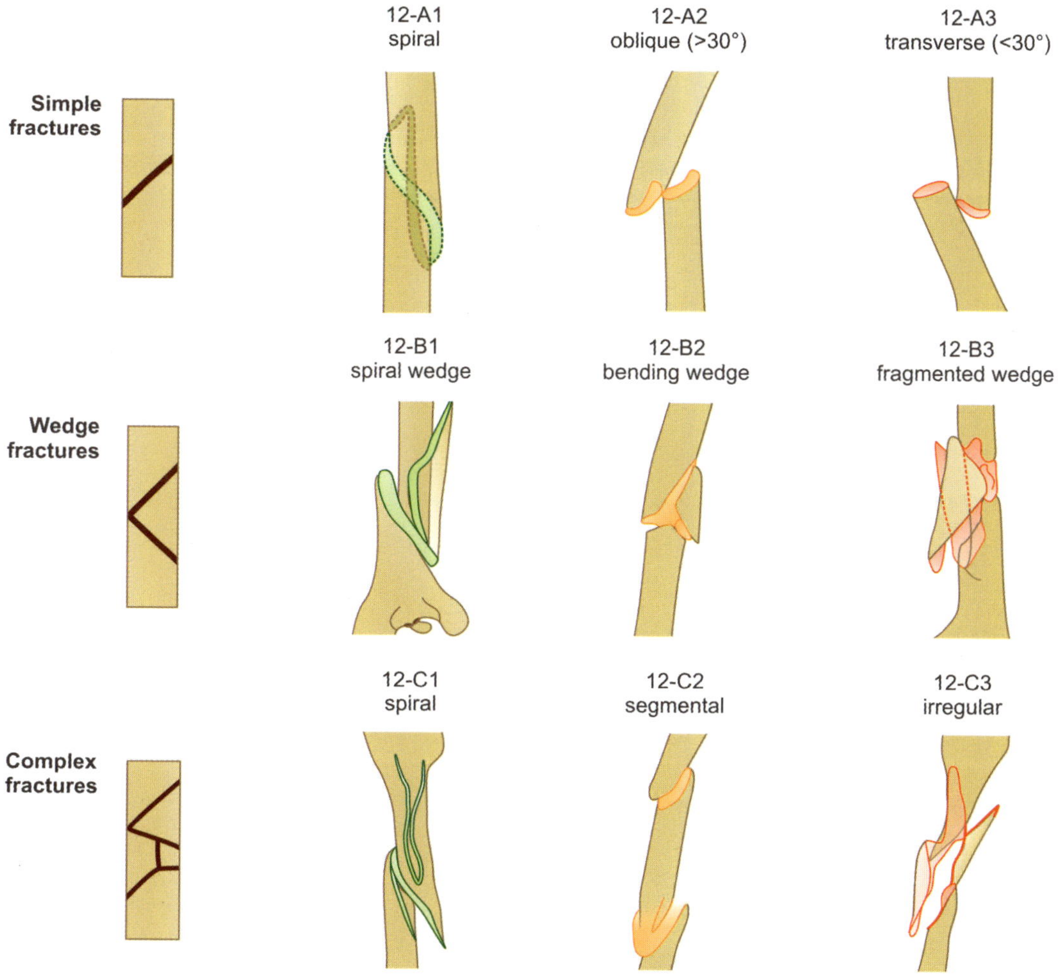

12-A1
spiral

12-A2
oblique (>30°)

12-A3
transverse (<30°)

Simple fractures

12-B1
spiral wedge

12-B2
bending wedge

12-B3
fragmented wedge

Wedge fractures

12-C1
spiral

12-C2
segmental

12-C3
irregular

Complex fractures

Fig. 3.9a: AO classification of humeral diaphyseal fractures.

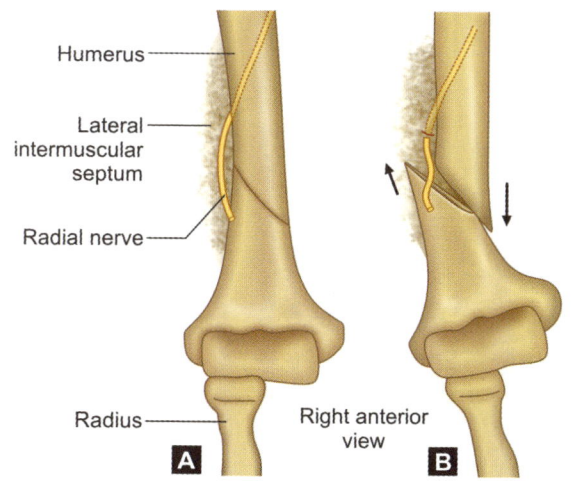

Humerus

Lateral intermuscular septum

Radial nerve

Radius

Right anterior view

A   B

Fig. 3.9b: Pictorial representation of Holstein and Lewis fracture and its relation with radial nerve.

10. DISTAL HUMERUS

AO/OTA Classification (Fig. 3.10a)

Humerus = 1, distal = 3.

Jupiter et al classification of 2-column distal humerus fracture (Fig. 3.10b): In Jupiter's model distal humerus is composed of two divergent columns that support an intercalary articular segment, which is similar to AO concept of condyles (Table 3.2).

Mehne and Matta et al Classification

It is also based on Jupiters model.

• *Intra-articular*: Bicolumn, unicolumnar and articular fractures.

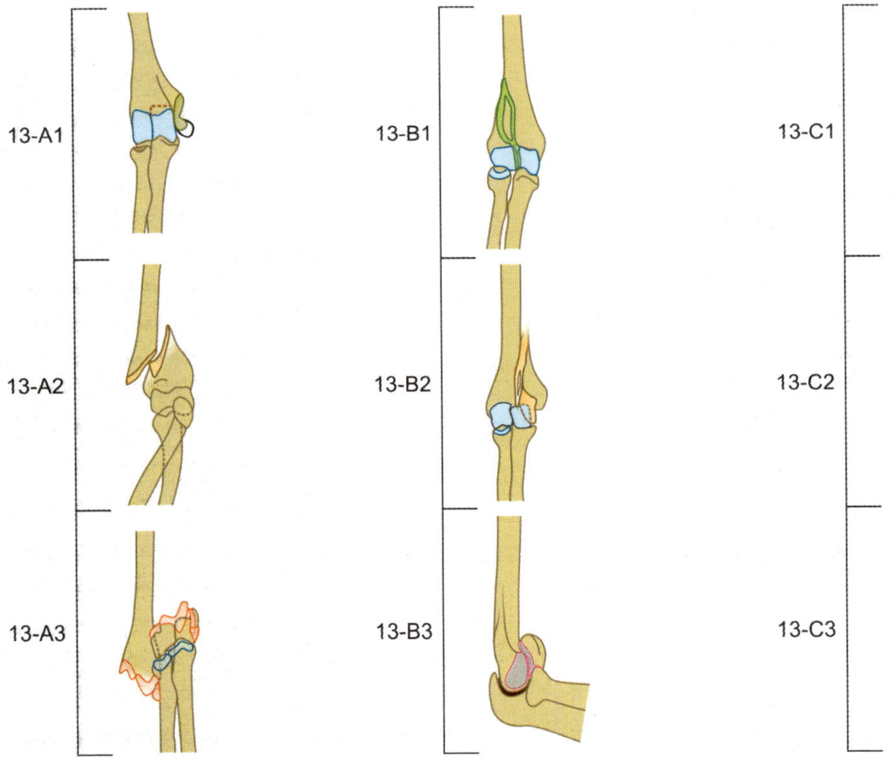

13-A1

13-B1

13-C1

13-A2

13-B2

13-C2

13-A3

13-B3

13-C3

13-A Extra-articular fracture	13-B Partial articular fracture	13-C Complete articular fracture
13-A1 Apophyseal avulsion	13-B1 Sagittal lateral condyle	13-C1 Articular simple, metaphyseal simple
13-A2 Metaphyseal simple	13-B2 Sagittal medial condyle	13-C2 Articular simple, metaphyseal multifragmentary
13-A3 Metaphyseal multifragmentary	13-B3 Coronal	13-C3 Articular multifragmentary

Fig. 3.10a: AO/OTA classification of distal humerus fracture.

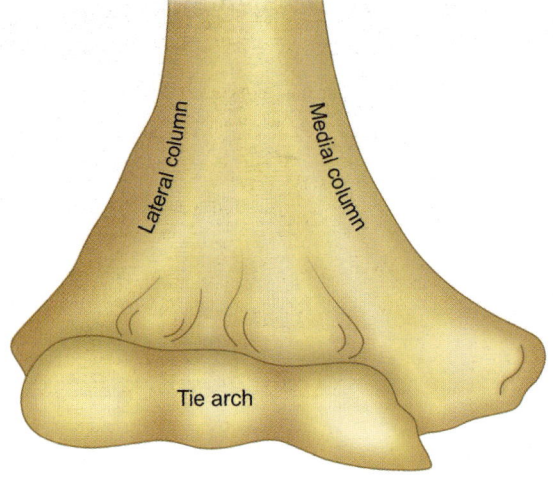

Fig. 3.10b: Jupiter's column concept of distal humerus.

TABLE 3.2: Jupiter classification of two-column distal humerus fracture	
High-T	Transverse fracture proximal to or at upper olecranon fossa
Low-T	Transverse fracture just proximal to trochlea (common)
Y	Oblique fracture line through both columns with distal vertical fx line
H	Trochlea is a free fragment (risk of AVN)
Medial lambda	Proximal fracture line exists medially
Lateral lambda	Proximal fracture line exists laterally
Multiplane T	T type with additional fracture in coronal plane

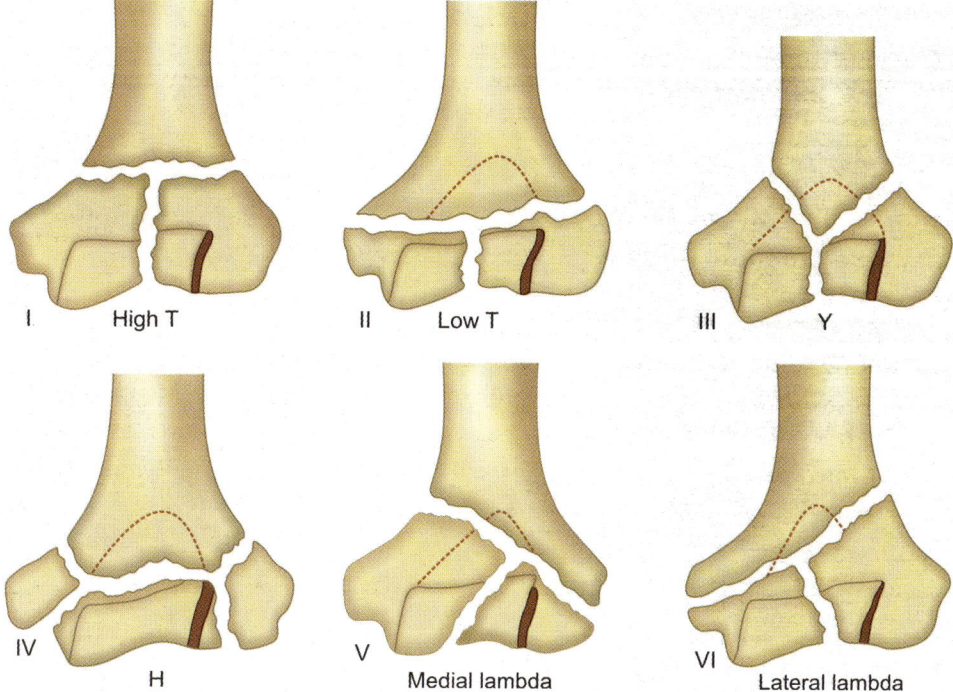

Fig. 3.10c: Jupiter's columnar concept of distal humerus fractures.

- *Extra-articular, intracapsular*: High/low trans-columnar.
- *Extra-capsular*: Medial/lateral epicondyle fracture.

11. INTERCONDYLAR FRACTURES

Riseborough and Radin Classification
(Fig. 3.11)

- *Type I.* Nondisplaced
- *Type II.* Slight displacement with no rotation between the condylar fragments in the frontal plane
- *Type III.* Displacement with rotation
- *Type IV.* Severe comminution of the articular surface.

12. CONDYLAR FRACTURES

Milch Classification (Fig. 3.12)

This system is based on whether the lateral portion of the trochlea remains attached to the humeral shaft.

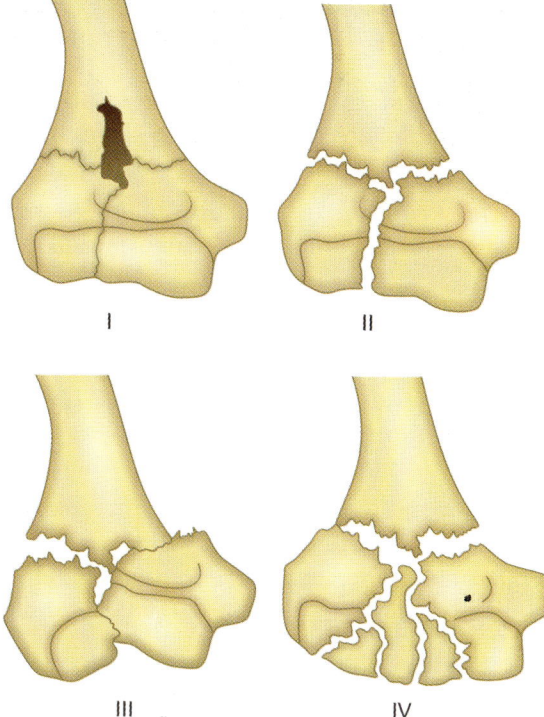

Fig. 3.11: Riseborough and Radin classification of distal humerus fracture.

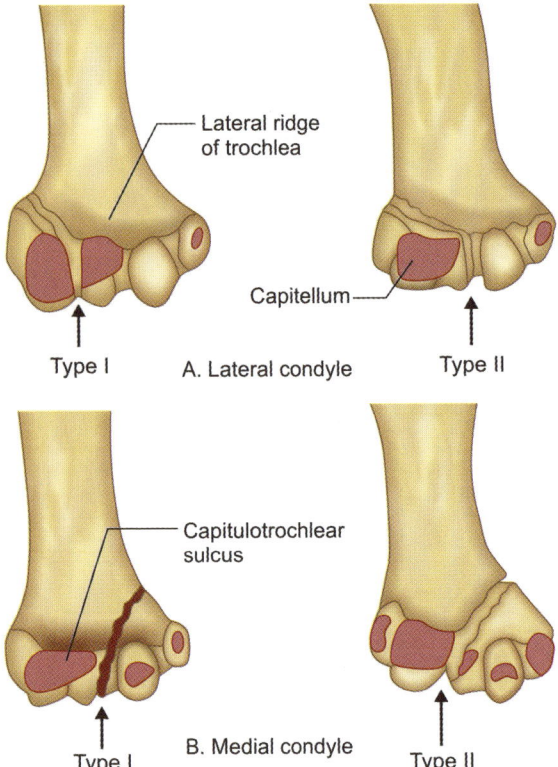

Fig. 3.12: Milch classification of condylar fractures of humerus.

Milch type I. The medial or lateral condyle can be fractured but the lateral eminence of trochlea remains attached to the humeral shaft. They are Salter Harris type IV fracture.

Milch type II. The lateral eminence of the trochlea is a part of the column fracture. They are Salter Harris type II fracture.

Type II fracture are unstable and may allow for radioulnar translocation if capsuloligamentous disruption occurs on the contralateral side.

Jackobs Classification

- *Stage I.* Undisplaced with intact articular surface (Badelon modification – displacement <2 mm)
- *Stage II.* Complete fracture through articular surface.

- *Stage III.* Fragment rotated, displaced laterally and proximally allowing translocation of olecranon and radial head.

Finnbogason and Associates Classification

They classified only minimally displaced fractures, i.e. ≤2 mm.

- *Type A.* Minimal/no gap on radial side/dorsal side. # not continuous to epiphyseal cartilage.
- *Type B.* As above but # line continuous to articular surface.
  Lateral # gap > medial.
- *Type C.* As of B but # gap as wide medially as laterally.

Weiss et al

- *Type I.* <2 mm displacement
- *Type II.* >2 m displacement
- *Type III.* >2 mm displacement but no intact articular surface.

13. CAPITELLUM FRACTURES

Classification (Fig. 3.13a)

- *Type I.* **Hahn-Steinthal I** fragment. Large osseous component of capitellum, sometimes with trochlear involvement.
- *Type II.* **Kocher-Lorenz fragment**. Articular cartilage with minimal subchondral bone attached: "uncapping of the condyle".
- *Type III.* Markedly comminuted (introduced by **Bryan and Morrey**).
- *Type IV.* Extension into trochlea (introduced by **Mcknee et al**—a type I fracture with medial extension to include the lateral half of trochlea also known as **Hahn-Steinthal II**).

Dubberly et al Classification (Fig. 3.13b)

For capitellar and trochlea fracture

- *Type I.* Fracture of capitellum with/without lateral trochlear ridge.
- *Type II.* Fracture involves capitellum and most of the trochlea as one piece.
- *Type III.* Capitellum and trochlea are separate pieces.

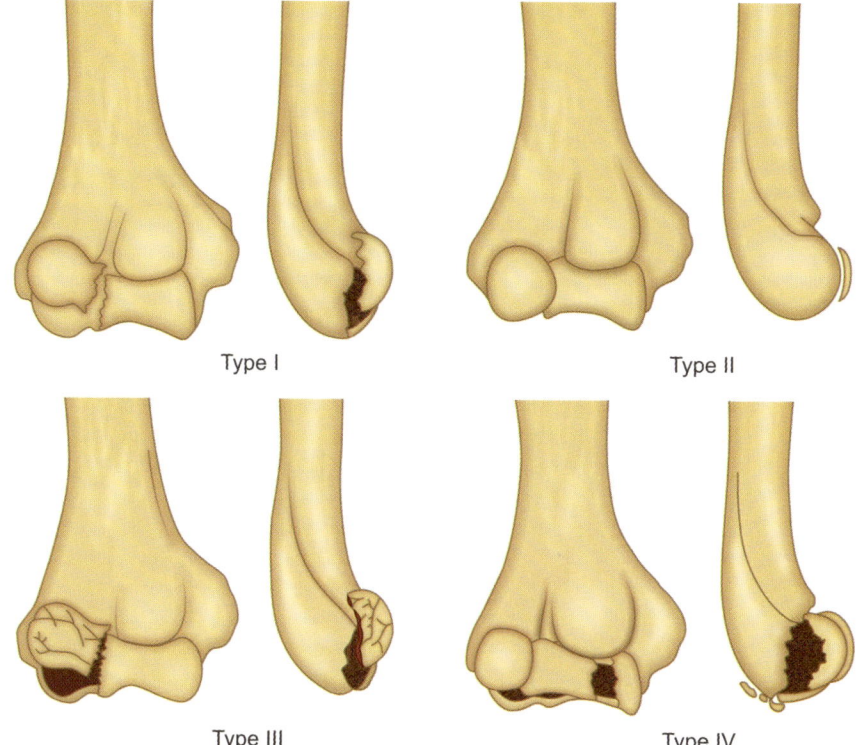

Type I   Type II

Type III   Type IV

Fig. 3.13a: Bryan and Morrey capitellum fracture classification.

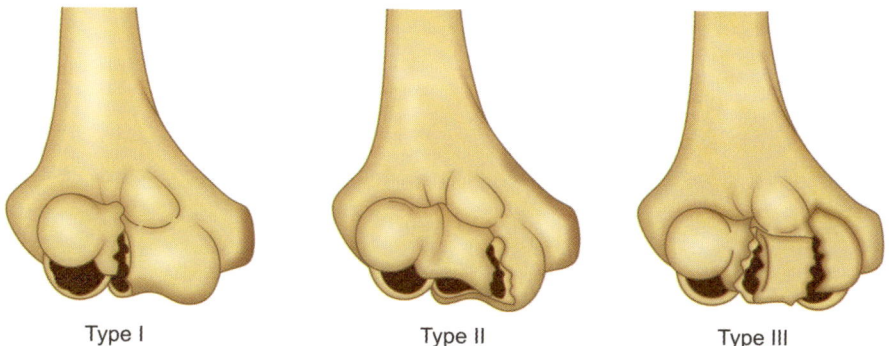

Type I   Type II   Type III

Fig. 3.13b: Dubberly et al classification for capitellar and trochlea fracture.

14. CORONOID PROCESS FRACTURE

Regan and Morrey Classification (Fig. 3.14a)

- *Type I.* Fracture avulsion just the tip of the coronoid.
- *Type II.* Those that involve less than 50% of coronoid either as single fracture or multiple fragments.
- *Type III.* Those involve >50% of coronoid.

Subdivided into those without (A) and with elbow dislocation (B).

O'Driscoll et al Classification (Fig. 3.14b)

Subdivides coronoid fracture based on location and number of coronoid fragment.

It also recognises anteromedial facet fracture caused by varus posteromedial rotational force.

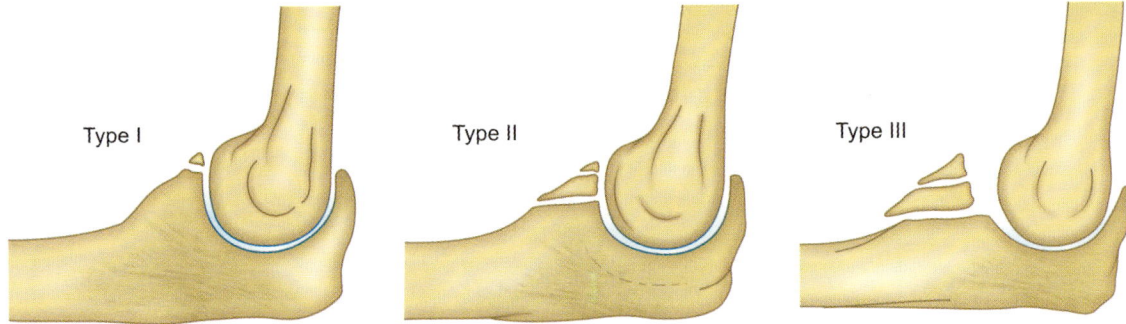

Fig. 3.14a: Regan and Morrey classification of coronoid process fracture.

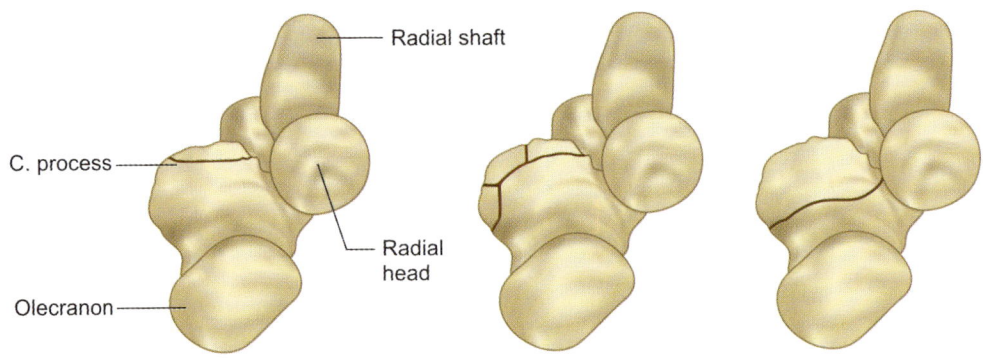

Fig. 3.14b: O'Driscoll et al classification for coronoid fractures.

Type I. Tip fractures

- Typically associated with fractures of radial head and a concomitant elbow dislocation, the terrible triad injury of the elbow. These injury occur with PLRI mechanism.
  - *Subtype 1.* ≤2 mm of coronoid height
  - *Subtype 2.* >2 mm of coronoid height, but less than 50% of coronoid height.

Type II. Anteromedial fractures

- These are seen with PMRI of elbow and are almost always have a concomitant avulsion of the LCL.
  - *Subtype 1.* Fracture of the anteromedial rim
  - *Subtype 2.* Fracture of the anteromedial rim and tip
  - *Subtype 3.* Fracture of the anteromedial rim and sublime tubercle with or without involvement of the tip.

Type III. Basal fractures

- M/C associated with injury of olecranon and proximal ulna and have a more direct posterior injury mechanism.
  - *Subtype 1.* Fracture of the coronoid body and base (at least 50% of the height of the coronoid)
  - *Subtype 2.* Includes the former associated with olecranon fractures.

15. OLECRANON FRACTURE

Mayo Classification

Based on comminution, displacement, fracture-dislocation (Fig. 3.15a)

- **Type I.** Undisplaced, stable fractures
- **Type II.** Displaced, elbow stable
- **Type III.** Displaced, unstable fractures

These are further subdivided into type A and B for noncomminuted and comminuted fractures.

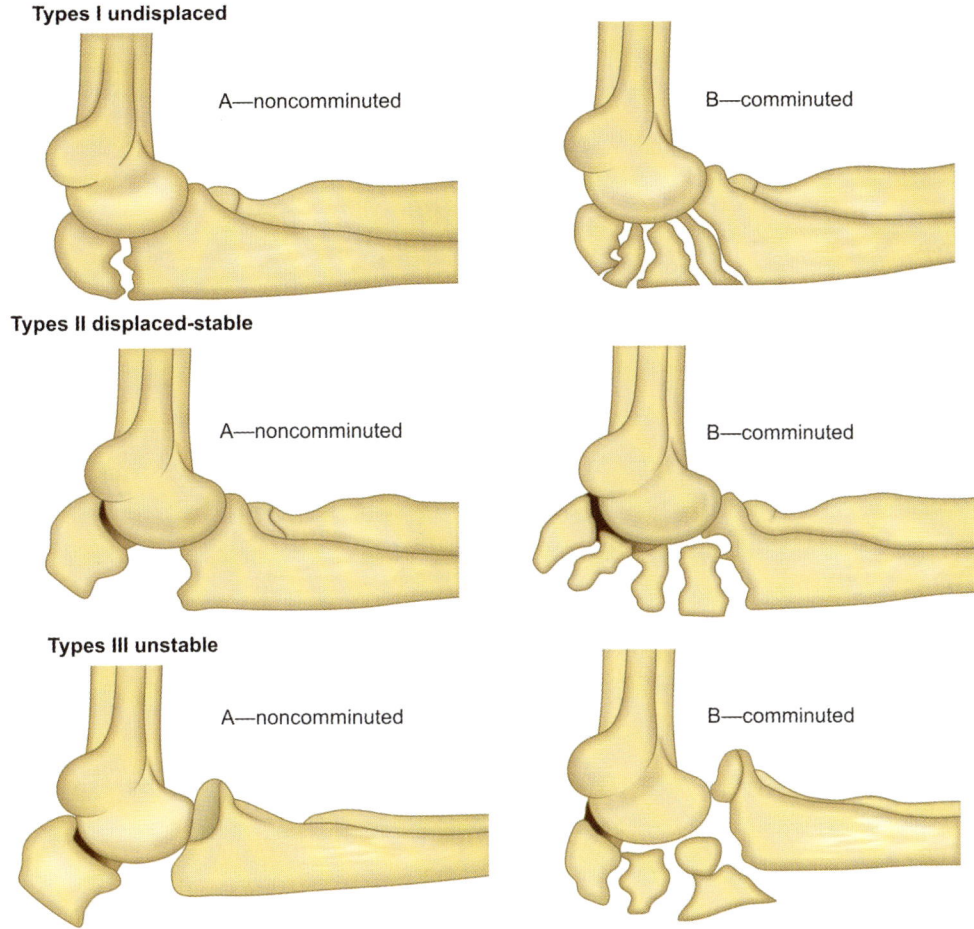

Fig. 3.15a: Mayo classification of olecranon fracture.

Colton Classification (Table 3.3)

TABLE 3.3: Colton classification of olecranon fractures (Fig. 3.15b)	
Nondisplaced or displacement less than 2 mm	Displacement does not increase with elbow flexion Elbow extensor mechanism remains intact
Displaced	**A.** Avulsion fractures
	B. Oblique or transverse fractures
	C. Comminuted
	D. Fracture dislocations

Schatzker Classification (Table 3.4)

TABLE 3.4: Schatzker classification (Fig. 3.15c)			
Type A	Simple transverse fracture	Type D	Comminuted fracture
Type B	Transverse impacted fracture	Type E	More distal fracture, extra-articular
Type C	Oblique fracture	Type F	Fracture-dislocation

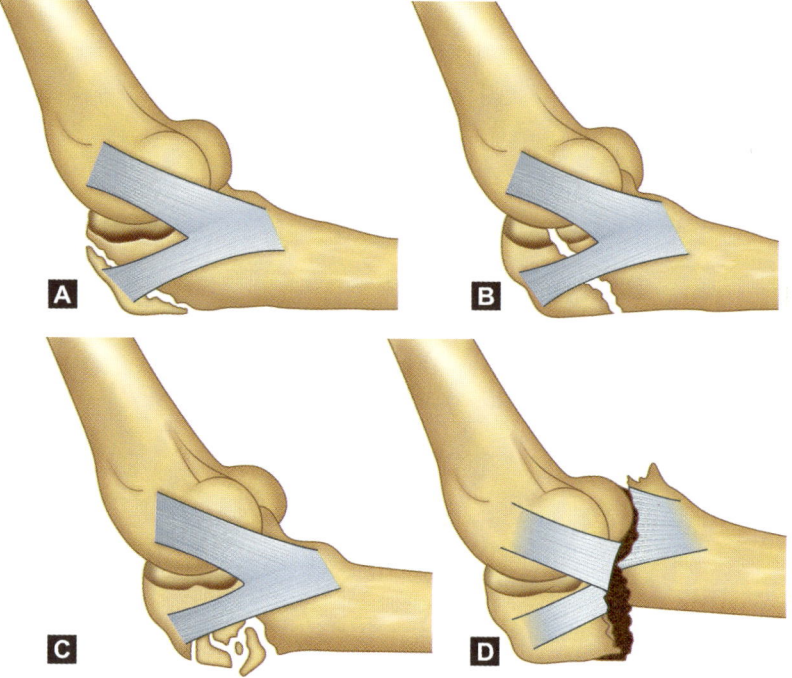

Fig. 3.15b: Colton classification of olecranon fractures.

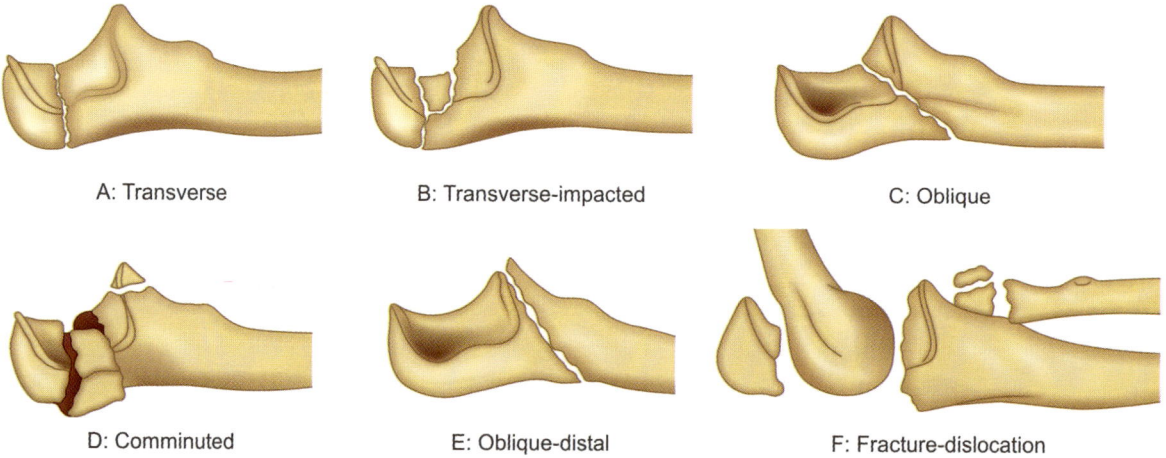

A: Transverse   B: Transverse-impacted   C: Oblique

D: Comminuted   E: Oblique-distal   F: Fracture-dislocation

Fig 3.15c: Schatzker classification of olecranon fracture.

16. RADIAL HEAD FRACTURE

Mason Classification (Fig. 3.16)

- *Type I.* Nondisplaced marginal fractures.
- *Type II.* Marginal fractures with displacement (impaction, depression, angulation).
- *Type III.* Comminuted fractures involving the entire head.

- *Type IV.* Associated with dislocation of the elbow (**Johnston** modification).

Broberg and Morrey Classification

Morrey modified the above classification and included radial neck # and quantified displacement.

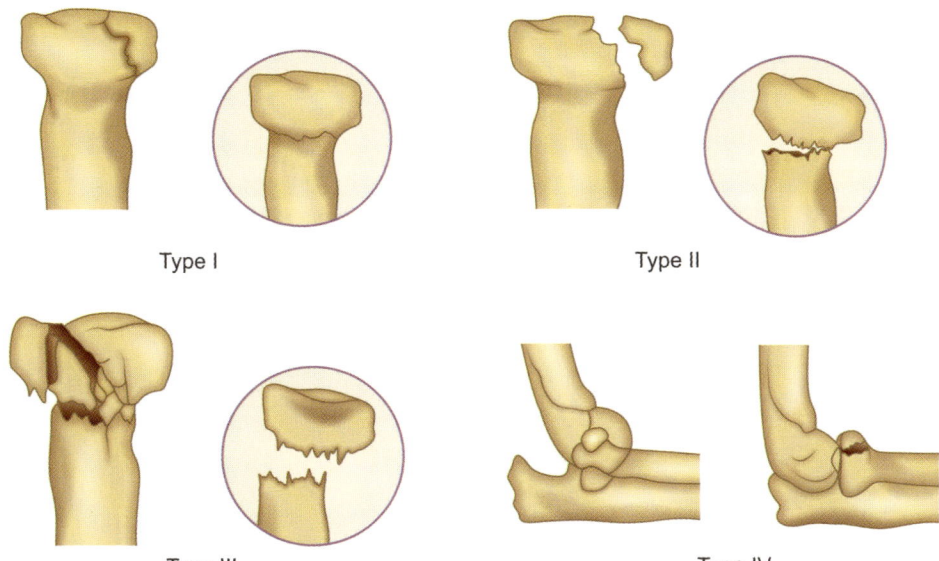

Fig. 3.16: Mason classification of radial head fracture.

- *Type I.* Fracture is undisplaced or displaced less than 2 mm and involves less than 30% of the articular surface area.
- *Type II.* Fracture is displaced more than 2 mm and involves more than 30% of the articular surface area.
- *Type III.* Fracture is comminuted.

Hotchkiss Modification

It reflects treatment option.
- *Type I.* Minimally displaced fracture. They do well with nonoperative treatment.
- *Type II.* Displaced partial head fracture that blocks forearm rotation and fracture involving the entire radial head that are irreparable.
- *Type III.* Irreperable fracture that require excision with/without prosthetic placement.

The Comprehensive Classification of Fracture

Mixes fracture of proximal radius and ulna, that are not useful for patient management. But it distinguishes fracture with more than 3 fragments from those having 2–3 major fragments. Fracture with more than 3 fragments has been associated with a much higher risk of failure of internal fixation, non-union and forearm rotation.

17. ELBOW DISLOCATION

Classification

- *Chronology*: Acute, chronic (unreduced), recurrent
- *Descriptive*: Based on relationship of radius/ulna to the distal humerus, as follows (Fig. 3.17):
  - Posterior
    - Posterolateral: >90% dislocations
    - Posteromedial
  - Anterior
  - Lateral
  - Medial
  - Divergent (rare)

18. FOREARM FRACTURE

A. AO/OTA Classification (Fig. 3.18a)

Forearm = 2, diaphysis = 2.

B. Monteggia Fracture

Fracture of the shaft of the ulna with associated dislocation of the proximal radioulnar joint.

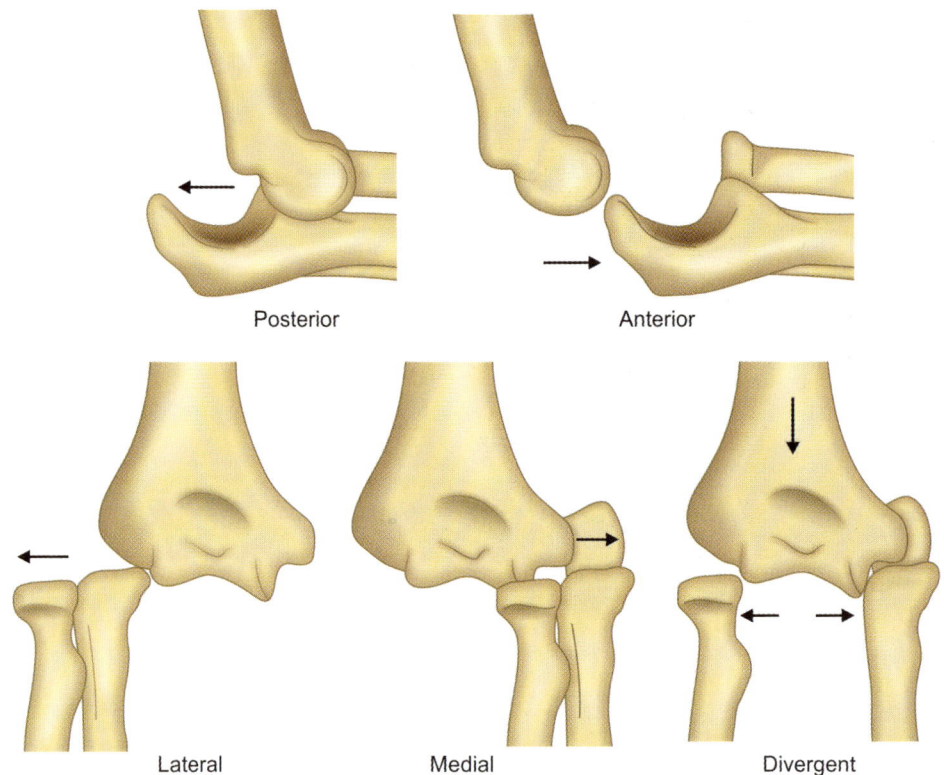

Posterior   Anterior

Lateral   Medial   Divergent

*Anterior–posterior type (ulna posterior, radial head anterior).
*Mediolateral (transverse) type (distal humerus wedged between radius lateral and ulna medial).

Fig. 3.17: Classification of elbow dislocation according to its direction of displacement.

22   Radius/Ulna diaphysis

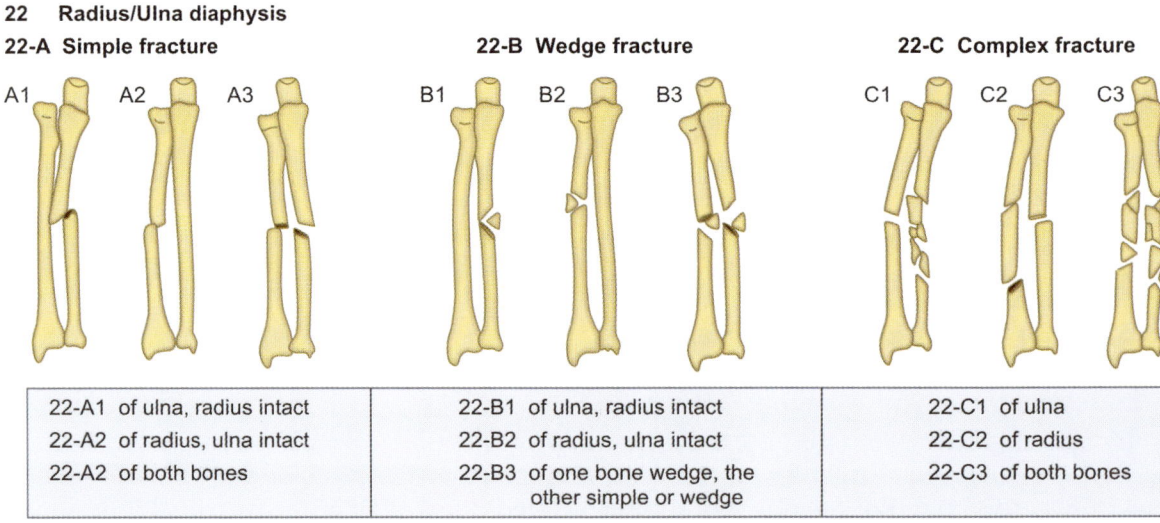

22-A Simple fracture	22-B Wedge fracture	22-C Complex fracture
A1 A2 A3	B1 B2 B3	C1 C2 C3

22-A1 of ulna, radius intact	22-B1 of ulna, radius intact	22-C1 of ulna
22-A2 of radius, ulna intact	22-B2 of radius, ulna intact	22-C2 of radius
22-A2 of both bones	22-B3 of one bone wedge, the other simple or wedge	22-C3 of both bones

Fig. 3.18a: AO/OTA classification of forearm fractures.

Bado Classification (Fig. 3.18b)

The classification is based on mechanism of injury and does not deal with treatment/prognosis.

- **Type I.** Anterior dislocation of the radial head with fracture of the ulnar diaphysis at any level with anterior angulation.
- **Type II.** Posterior/posterolateral dislocation of the radial head with fracture of the ulnar diaphysis with posterior angulation.
- **Type III.** Lateral/anterolateral dislocation of the radial head with fracture of the ulnar metaphysis. This occurs almost exclusively in children, but isolated cases in adults have been described.
- **Type IV.** Anterior dislocation of the radial head with fractures of both the radius and ulna within proximal third at the same level. This occurs almost exclusively in adult patients.

Jupiter et al, further subdivided Bado's Type II into:

IIA. Ulnar # involving coronoid process and olecranon.

IIB. # distal to coronoid at the junction of metaphysis–diaphysis.

IIC. Ulnar # strictly diaphyseal.

IID. Complex pattern of ulna # from olecranon to ulna diaphysis.

Monteggia Equivalents

Type I

- Isolated dislocation of radial head.
- Radial neck fracture (isolated).
- Radial neck fracture in combination with a fracture of the ulnar diaphysis.
- Radial and ulnar fractures with the radial fracture above the junction of the middle and proximal thirds.

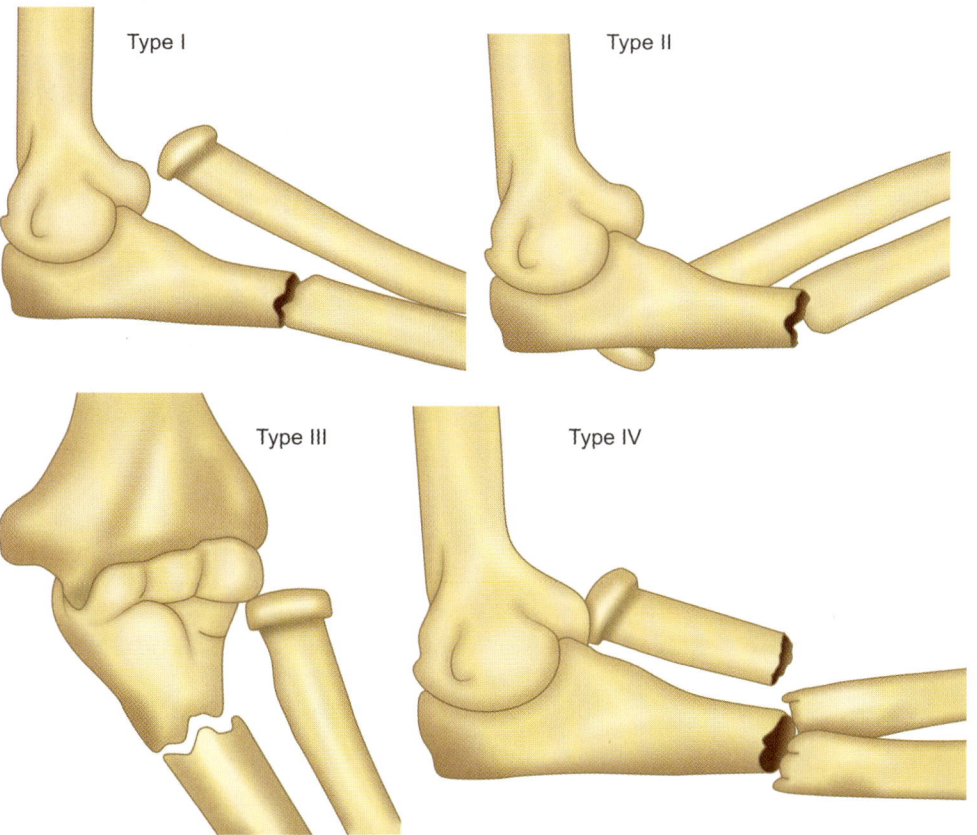

Fig. 3.18b: Bado classification.

- Fracture of ulnar diaphysis with anterior displocation of radial head and an olecranon fracture.

Type II

- Posterior dislocation of the elbow.
- Posterior dislocation of radial head associated with fracture of radial epiphysis/neck.

Type III. Described by **Ravessoud**

- An oblique fracture of the ulna with varus alignment and a displaced lateral condylar fracture.

Type IV. Described by **Arazi**

- Fracture of the distal humerus with ulnar diaphysis fracture and fracture of radial neck.
    1. Anterior dislocation of the radial head with plastic deformation of the ulna.
    2. Fracture of the ulnar diaphysis with a fracture of the neck of the radius.
    3. Fracture of the ulnar diaphysis with a fracture of the proximal third of the radius proximal to the ulnar fracture.
    4. Fracture of the ulnar metaphysis with anterior dislocation of the radius.
    5. Fracture of the ulnar diaphysis with anterior dislocation of the radial head and fracture of the olecranon.
    6. Fracture of the ulnar metaphysis with fracture of the neck of the radius.
    7. Posterior dislocation of the elbow and fracture of the ulnar diaphysis, with or without fracture of the proximal radius.

C. Galeazzi Fracture (Fig. 3.18c)

Fracture of the radial shaft with dislocation of the distal radioulnar joint. They are subclassified according to the distance of the radial fracture from the articular surface.

- **Type I.** Occur within 7.5 cm of the articular surface of the distal radius.
    - Ulnar head anteriorly dislocated more commonly.
- **Type II.** They occur proximally
    - Ulnar head posteriorly dislocated.

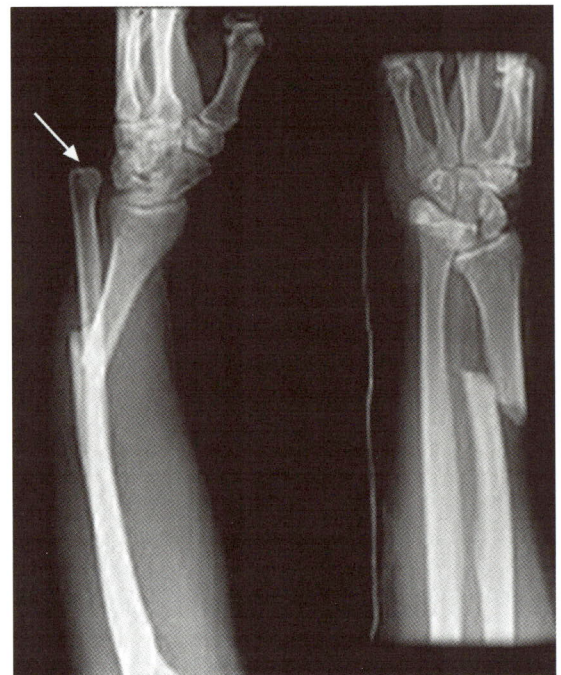

Fig. 3.18c: X-ray of Galeazzi fracture.

Variant: In children separation of DRUJ occurs through a displaced Salter Harris type II physeal fracture of distal ulna. However, in adult DRUJ dislocation cannot occur without disruption of the triangular fibrocartilagenous complex, but in children with open physis, the distal ulnar physis can avulse before rupture of the complex and interposition of the periosteum may block rotation.

19. DISTAL RADIUS FRACTURE

A. Gartland and Werley Classification (Fig. 3.19a)

- **Group I.** Simple Colles' fracture with no involvement of the radial articular surfaces
- **Group II.** Comminuted Colles' fractures with intra-articular extension without displacement
- **Group III.** Comminuted Colles' fractures with intra-articular extension with displacement
- **Group IV.** Extra-articular, undisplaced (Solgaard modification).

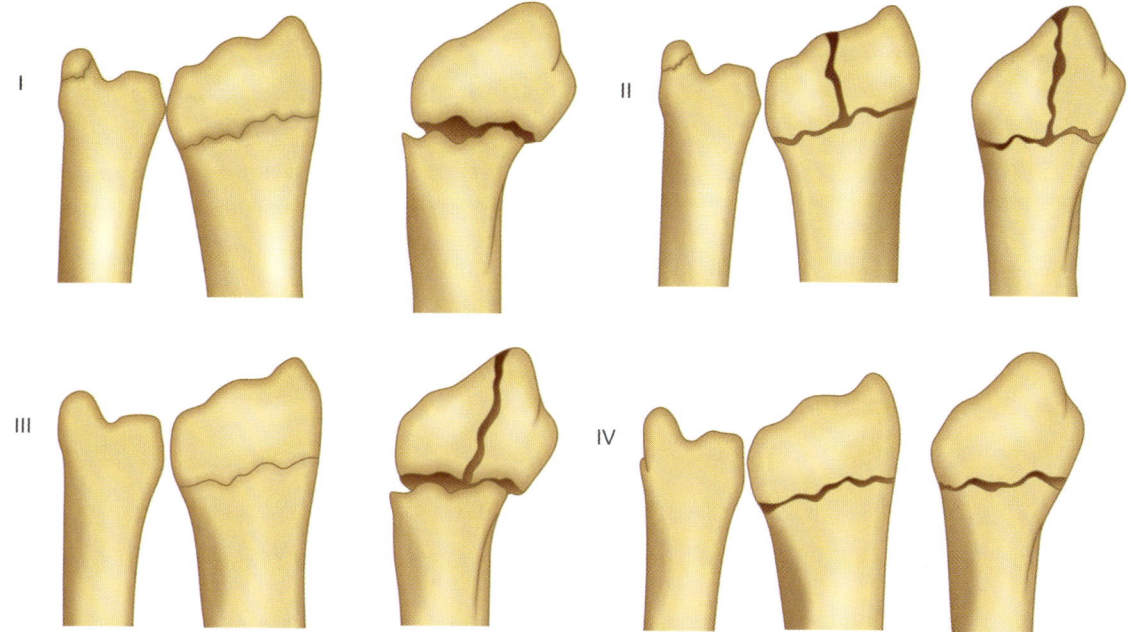

Fig. 3.19a: Gartland and Werley classification of distal radius fracture.

B. Frykman Classification (Fig. 3.19b)

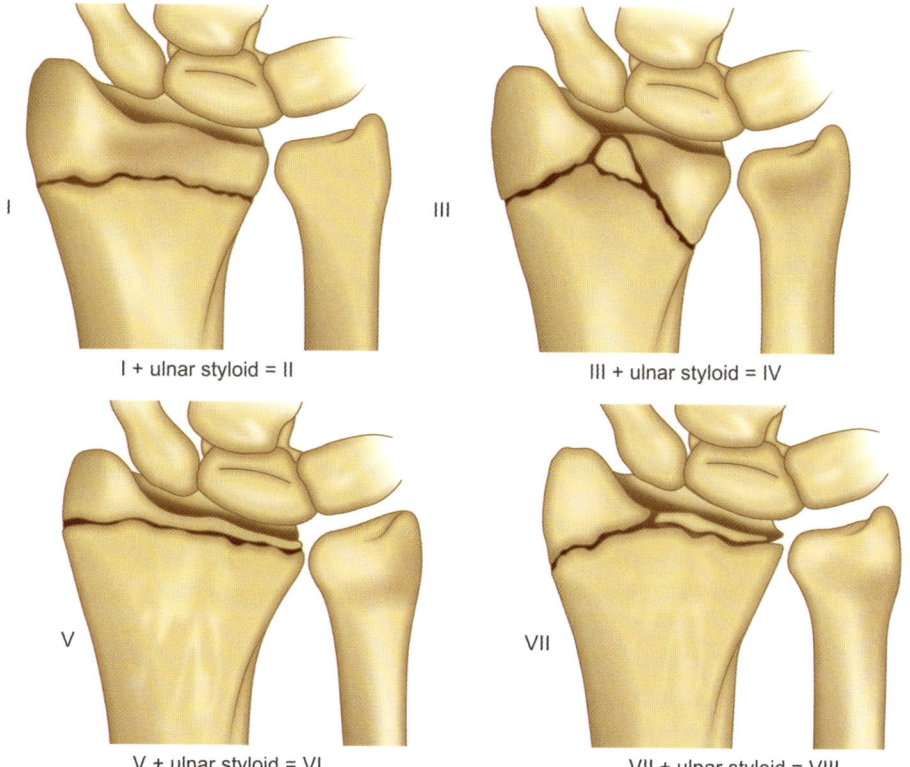

I + ulnar styloid = II

III + ulnar styloid = IV

V + ulnar styloid = VI

VII + ulnar styloid = VIII

Fig. 3.19b: Frykman classification.

C. Melone Classification

Melone classified intra-articular fractures of distal radius by considering that each fragment consisted of four parts—radial styloid, dorsal medial fragment, volar medial fragment, and the radial shaft (Fig. 3.19c1). He termed the two medial fragments which make-up the lunate fossa the medial complex and based his classification based on the position of medial complex (Table 3.5 and Fig. 3.19c2).

D. Cooney (Universal) Classification (Fig. 3.19d)

- *Type I.* Extra-articular, undisplaced
- *Type II.* Extra-articular, displaced
  - IIA. Reducible and stable
  - IIB. Reducible and unstable
  - IIC. Irreducible.
- *Type III.* Intra-articular, undisplaced
- **Type IV.** Intra-articular, displaced
  - IVA. Reducible and stable
  - IVB. Reducible and unstable
  - IVC. Irreducible.

TABLE 3.5: Melone classification of DER fracture

Type	Description
Type I	**Undisplaced** fracture with no or minimal comminution
Type II	**Unstable "die punch"** fracture with moderate to severe displacement of the medial complex as a unit with comminution of the dorsal and volar cortex • **Type IIa:** Reducible • **Type IIb:** Irreducible, because of impaction
Type III	Fracture with **spike fragment** of the radius on the volar side—commonly associated with median nerve or tendon injury
Type IV	**Split fracture, unstable.** The medial complex fragments are severely comminuted with rotation of the fragments
Type V	**Explosion fracture** with severe comminution, transverse split, and rotational displacement

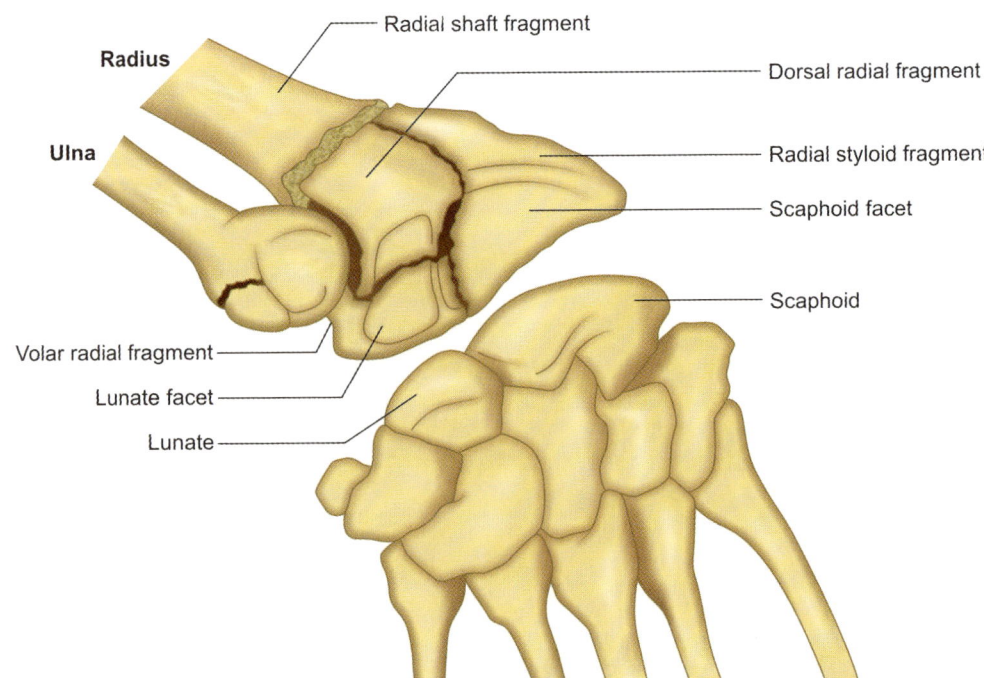

Fig. 3.19c1: Normal anatomy of distal end radius with wrist joint.

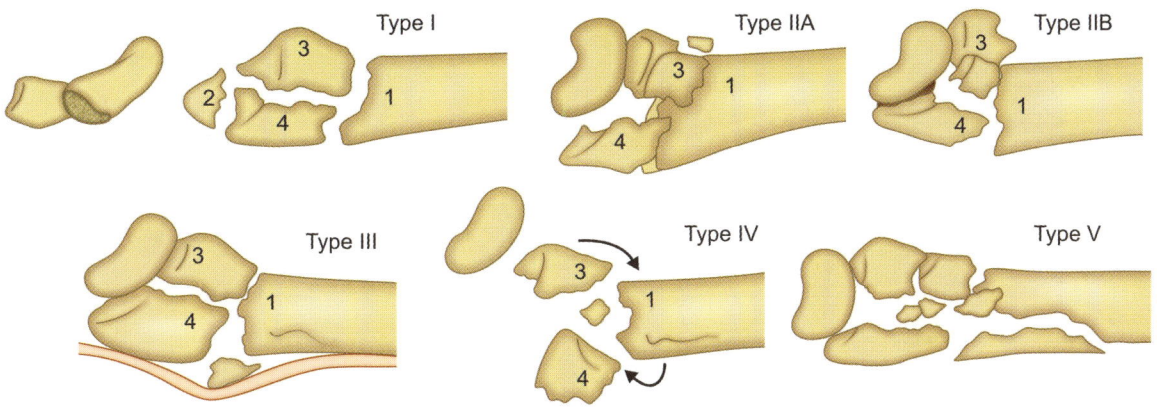

Fig. 3.19c2: Melone classification of DER fracture.

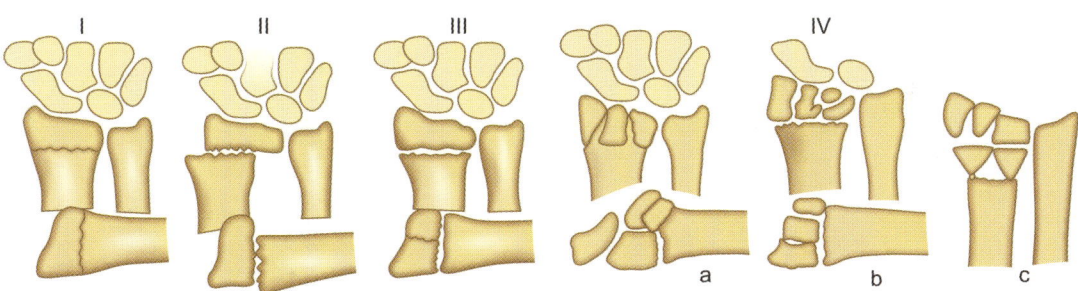

Fig. 3.19d: Cooney (universal) classification of DER fracture.

E. Fernandez Classification (Table 3.6)

TABLE 3.6: Fernandez classification (Fig. 3.19e)	
I. Bending	Metaphyseal bending fractures with the inherent problems of loss of palmar tilt and radial shortening relative to the ulna (DRUJ injuries). One cortex of the metaphysis fails due to tensile stress (Colles' and Smith fractures), and the opposite cortex undergoes some comminution
II. Shearing	Fracture of the joint surface: Barton's; reversed Barton's styloid process fracture, simple articular fracture. Shearing fractures requiring reduction and often buttressing of the articular segment
III. Compression	Fracture of the surface of the joint with impaction of subchondral and metaphyseal bone (die-punch); intra-articular comminuted fracture
IV. Avulsion	Fracture of the ligament attachments to ulnar and radial styloid process; radiocarpal fracture-dislocation
V. Combinations	Combination of types; high energy injuries

F. Modified AO Classification

- **Type A.** Extra-articular fracture. Subgroups are based upon angulation and comminution.
- **Type B.** Partial articular fracture
  B1. Radial styloid fracture
  B2. Dorsal rim fracture
  B3. Volar rim fracture
  B4. Die punch fracture.
- **Type C.** Complete articular. Subgroups are based on the articular surface's degree of comminution and the metaphysis.

G. Smith Fracture

Modified Thomas' classification (Fig. 3.19f)
- **Type A.** Extra-articular
- **Type B.** Fracture line crosses into the dorsal articular surface
- **Type C.** Fracture line enters the carpal joint (Volar Barton).

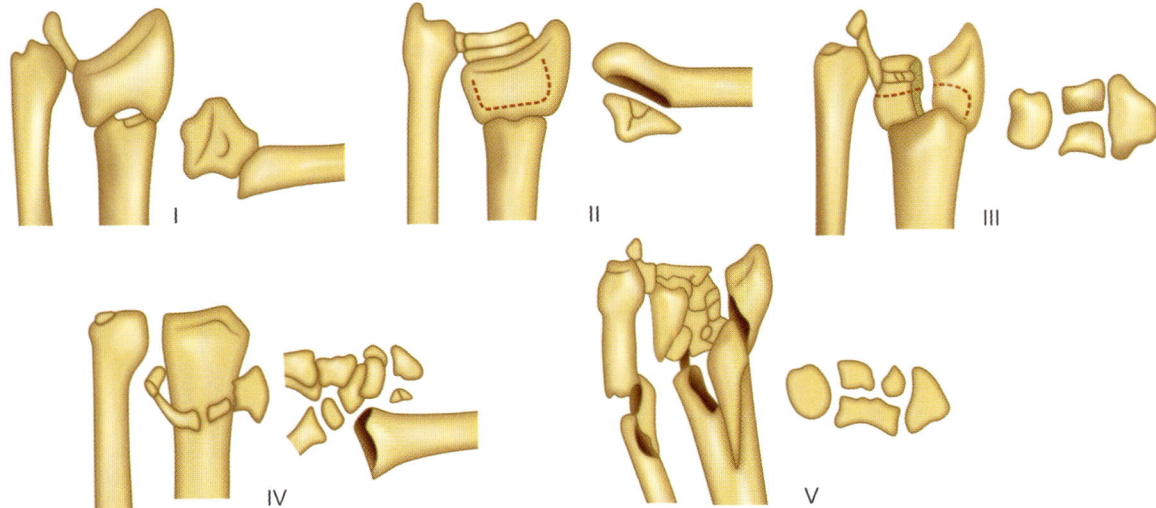

Fig. 3.19e: Fernandez classification of DER fracture.

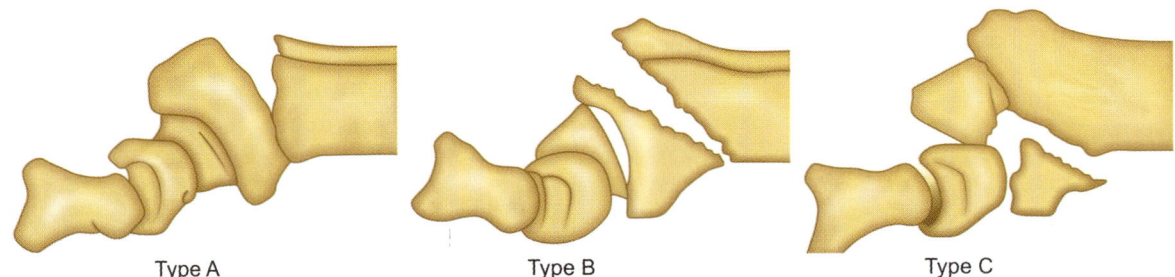

Fig. 3.19f: Modified Thomas' classification for Smith fracture.

20. SCAPHOID FRACTURES

A. Russe Classification (Fig. 3.20a)

1. Horizontal oblique
   - Distal third
   - Middle third (waist)
   - Proximal third
2. Transverse fracture line
3. Vertical oblique fracture line

B. Herbert and Fischer Classification (Fig. 3.20b)

- **Type A.** Acute stable fractures
  Type A1. Fracture of tubercle
  Type A2. Undisplaced "crack" fracture of the waist
- **Type B.** Acute unstable fractures
  Type B1. Oblique fractures of distal third
  Type B2. Displaced or mobile fracture of the waist

Type B3. Proximal pole fractures
Type B4. Fracture dislocation of carpus
Type B5. Comminuted fractures
- **Type C.** Delayed union
- **Type D.** Established nonunion
  Type D1. Fibrous non-union
  Type D2. Sclerotic nonunion (pseudoarthrosis).

21. LUNATE FRACTURES

Teisen and Hjarkbaek Classification (Fig. 3.21)

Group I. Fracture volar pole, possibly affecting the volar nutrient artery.

Group II. Chip fracture which does not affect the main blood supply.

Group III. Fracture of dorsal pole of the lunate possibly affecting the blood supply.

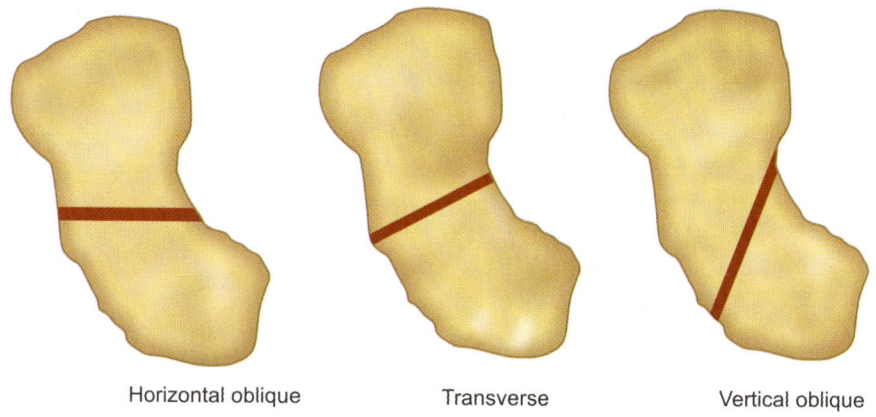

Horizontal oblique   Transverse   Vertical oblique

Fig. 3.20a: Russe classification of scaphoid fracture.

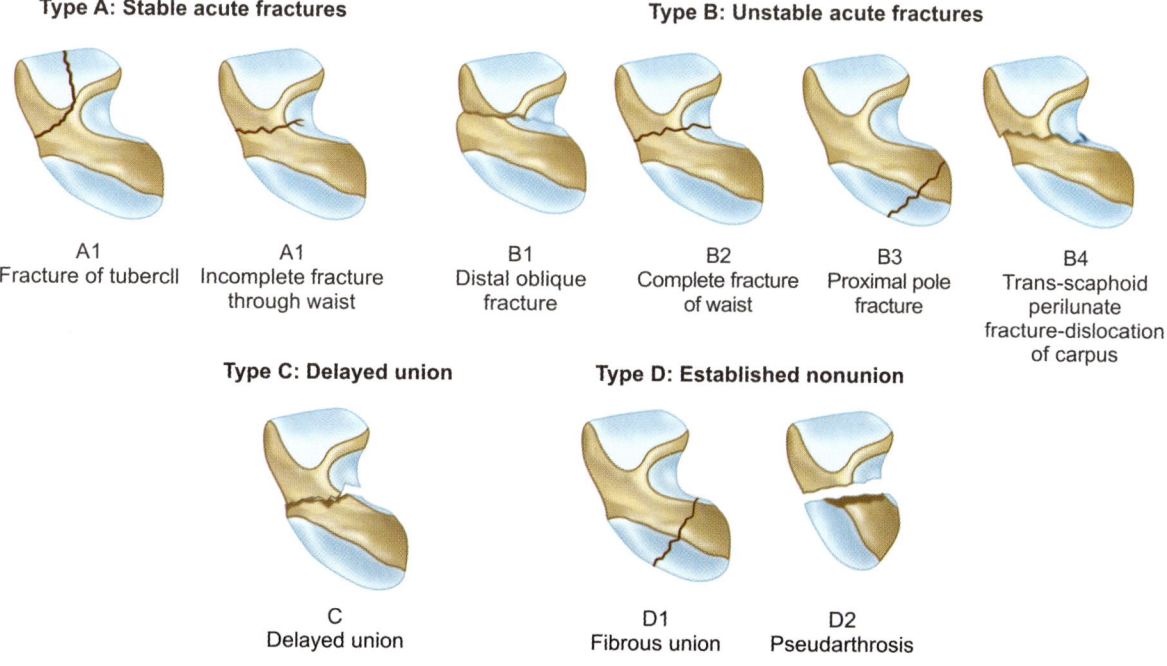

Type A: Stable acute fractures   **Type B: Unstable acute fractures**

| A1 | A1 | B1 | B2 | B3 | B4 |
| Fracture of tubercll | Incomplete fracture through waist | Distal oblique fracture | Complete fracture of waist | Proximal pole fracture | Trans-scaphoid perilunate fracture-dislocation of carpus |

Type C: Delayed union   **Type D: Established nonunion**

| C | D1 | D2 |
| Delayed union | Fibrous union | Pseudarthrosis |

Fig. 3.20b: Herbert and Fischer classification of scaphoid fracture.

Group IV. Sagittal fracture through the body of Lunate.

Group V. Transverse fractures through the body of the lunate.

22. THUMB

Intra-articular Fractures (Fig. 3.22)

- *Type I.* Bennett's fracture—fracture line separates major part of metacarpal from volar lip fragment, producing a disruption of the first carpometacarpal joint; first metacarpal is pulled proximally by the abductor pollicis longus.

- *Type II.* Rolando fracture—requires greater force than a Bennett fracture; presently used to describe a comminuted Bennett's fracture, a "Y" or "T" fracture, or a fracture with dorsal and palmar fragments.

Teisen classification	Anteroposterior view	Lateral view	Type
I			Volar pole
II			Chip fracture
III			Dorsal pole
IV			Sagittal
V			Transverse

Fig. 3.21: Teisen and Hjarkbaek classification of lunate fracture.

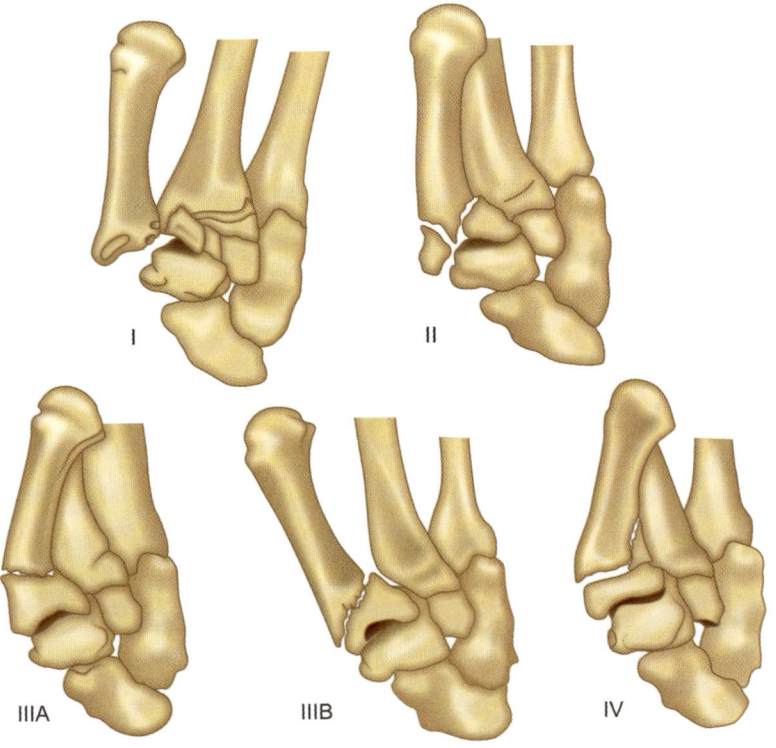

Fig. 3.22: Fracture classification of thumb.

Extra-articular Fractures

- *Type IIIA.* Transverse fracture
- *Type IIIB.* Oblique fracture
- *Type IV.* Epiphyseal injuries seen in children.

23. DISTAL PHALANX FRACTURES

A. Kaplan Classification

- *Type I.* Longitudinal split
- *Type II.* Comminuted tuft
- *Type III.* Transverse fracture

B. Mallet Fracture

Wehbe and Schneider Classification (Fig. 3.23)

- *Type I.* Mallet fractures including bone injuries of varying extent without sub-luxation of distal interphalangeal joint
- *Type II.* Fractures are associated with subluxation distal interphalangeal joint
- *Type III.* Epiphyseal and physeal injuries. Each type then divided into three subtypes:
  - *Type IIIA.* Fracture fragment involving less than one third of articular surface of distal phalanx
  - *Type IIIB.* A fracture fragment involving one-third to two-thirds of articular surface
- *Type IIIC.* A fragment that involves more than two-thirds of articular surface.

Mallet fingers are also classified into four types according to associated soft tissue injuries and the fracture pattern:

Type 1. Closed or blunt trauma with loss of tendon continuity with or without a small avulsion fracture

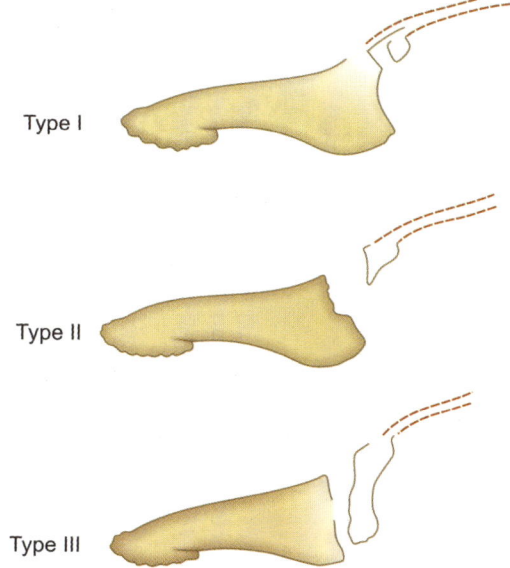

Fig. 3.23: Wehbe and Schneider classification.

Type 2. Laceration at or proximal to the distal interphalangeal joint with loss of tendon continuity

Type 3. Deep abrasion with loss of skin, sub-cutaneous cover, and tendon substance.

Type 4

- 4A—transphyseal fracture in children;
- 4B—hyperflexion injury with fracture of articular surface of 20 to 50%;
- 4C—hyperextension injury with fracture of the articular surface usually greater than 50% with early or late volar subluxation of the distal phalanx.

Type 1 mallet fingers are the most common.

Pelvis and Lower Limb

1. PELVIC FRACTURES

- Letournel
- Bucholz
- Tile
- Young and Burgess
- OTA/AO-research

Commonly used classification are Tile and Young and Burgess.

A. MODIFIED TILE CLASSIFICATION

Tile classification is a modification of Pennal Idea and they added the concept of stability.

The Tile classification system is mainly based on the integrity of the posterior sacro-iliac complex.

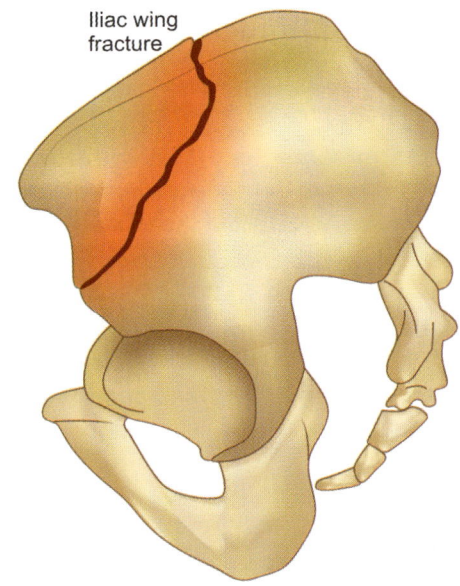

Fig. 4.1: Iliac wing fracture, classified as Tile type A1.

Tile Type A Fractures

- The SI joint is completely stable (rotationally and vertically)
- Fractures are outside the pelvic ring.

A. Stable

A1. Fracture not involving the ring (avulsion or iliac wing fracture) (Fig. 4.1).

A2. Stable or minimally displaced fracture of the ring.

A3. Transverse sacral fracture (Denis zone III sacral fracture).

Tile Type B Fractures

- Partial instability of the SI joint complex
- Rotationally unstable while vertically stable

B. Rotationally Unstable, Vertically Stable

B1. Open book injury (external rotation) (Fig. 4.2).

B2. Lateral compression injury (internal rotation)

- B2-1. With anterior ring rotation/displacement through ipsilateral rami

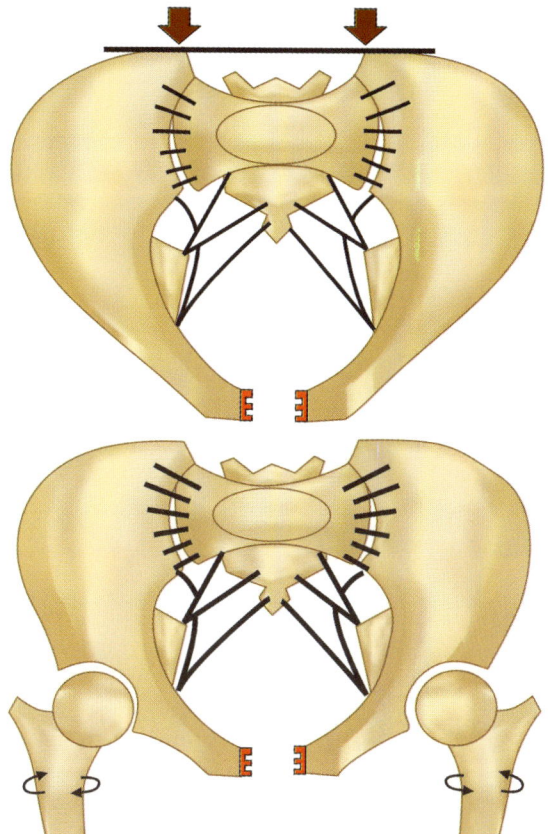

Fig. 4.2: Tile type B1, open book injury (external rotation).

- B2-2. With anterior ring rotation/displacement through contralateral rami (bucket-handle injury) (Fig. 4. 3)

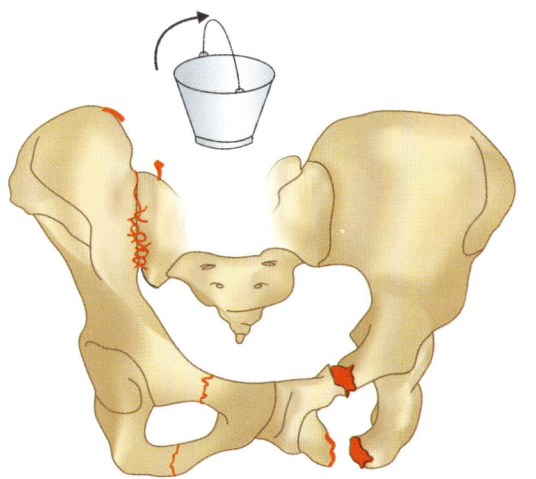

Fig. 4.3: Tile type B2-2, bucket handle injury.

B3. Bilateral type B fracture
- B3.1. Bilateral open book fracture
- B3.2. Open book fracture and lateral compression
- B3.3. Bilateral lateral compression

Type C Injuries—Unstable

Rotationally and vertically unstable, complete disruption of posterior arch.

C1. Unilateral
- C1-1. Iliac fracture
- C1-2. Sacroiliac fracture-dislocation
- C1-3. Sacral fracture

C2. Bilateral with one side type B and one side type C.

C3. Bilateral with both sides type C.

B. YOUNG AND BURGESS CLASSIFICATION

Young and Burgess classification is the original work of Pennal and based on the direction of forces causing fracture, associated instability of pelvis.

Four patterns of injury are described (Fig. 4.4):
1. Lateral compression
2. Anteroposterior compression
3. Vertical shear
4. Combined mechanical

Description

1. *Lateral compression (LC).* Transverse fractures of the pubic rami, ipsilateral, or contralateral to posterior injury.
- *LC type I.* Sacral compression on the side of impact.
- *LC type II.* Posterior iliac wing fracture (crescent) on the side of impact.
- *LC type III.* LC I or LC II injury on the side of impact; contralateral open book injury.

2. *Anteroposterior compression.* Symphyseal diastasis or longitudinal rami fractures.
- *APC type I.* <2.5 cm of symphyseal diastasis; vertical fractures of one or both pubic rami intact posterior ligaments.

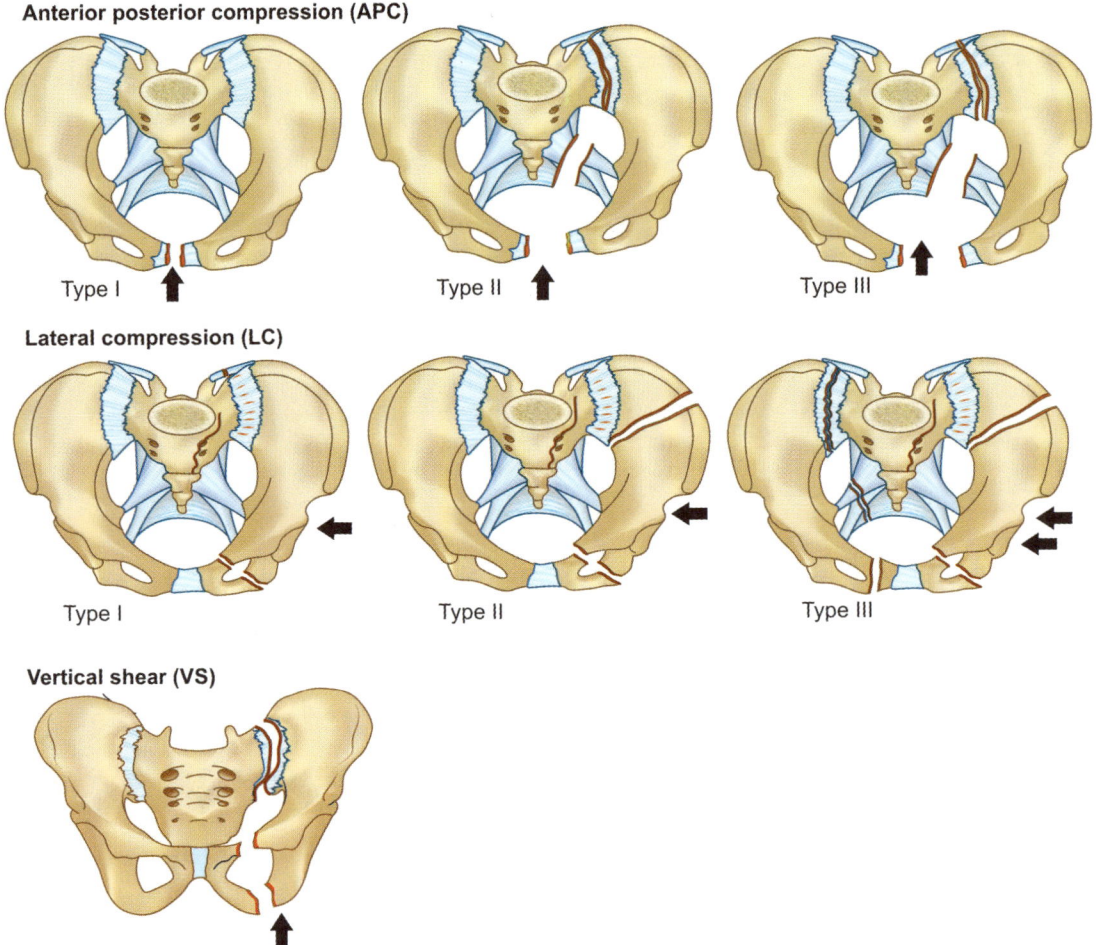

Fig. 4.4: Young and Burgess classification.

- *APC type II.* <2.5 cm of symphyseal diastasis; widening of sacroiliac joint due to anterior sacroiliac ligament disruption; disruption of the sacrotuberous, sacrospinous, and symphyseal ligaments with intact posterior sacroiliac ligaments result in "open book" injury with internal and external rotational instability; vertical stability is maintained.

- *APC type III.* Complete disruption of the symphysis, sacrotuberous, sacrospinous, and sacroiliac ligaments resulting in extreme rotational instability and lateral displacement; no cephaloposterior displacement; completely unstable with the highest rate of associated neurovascular injuries and blood loss.

3. *Vertical shears.* Symphyseal diastasis or vertical displaced anterior and posterior usually through the SI joint, occasionally through the iliac wing or sacrum.

4. *Combined mechanical.* Combination of injuries often due to crush mechanisms; most common is vertical shear and lateral compression.

- Tile and Young and Burgess classifications are the most commonly used classifications.
- Young and Burgess seems to be more easily remembered and reproduced.
- The prognostic values of both are comparable.
- Certain fractures may not be classifiable in either systems.

C. OPEN PELVIC FRACTURES

Jones Classification

Class 1: Stable open pelvic ring fractures (low mortality).

Class 2: Unstable open pelvic ring fractures without rectal injury (about 33% mortality).

Class 3: Unstable open pelvic ring fractures in combination with rectal injury (up to 50% mortality).

D. TORODE AND ZIEG CLASSIFICATION (Fig. 4.5)

Pediatric fracture classification.

Type I. Avulsion fractures

Type II. Iliac wing fractures

Type III. Simple pelvic ring fractures

Type IV. Pelvic ring disruption fractures

2. CLASSIFICATION OF ACETABULUM FRACTURE

Understanding acetabulum and its anatomical landmarks in radiology: This articular socket is composed of and supported by two columns of bone, described by Letournel and Judet as an inverted Y. The anterior column is composed of the anterior half of the iliac crest, the iliac spines, the anterior half of the acetabulum, and the pubis. The posterior column is the ischium, the ischial spine, the posterior half of the acetabulum, and the dense bone forming the sciatic notch. The posterior column begins at the superior aspect of the greater sciatic notch and is contiguous with the greater and lesser sciatic notches inferiorly and includes the ischial tuberosity. The anterior and posterior walls of the acetabulum are the components of the respective columns (Fig. 4.6a and b).

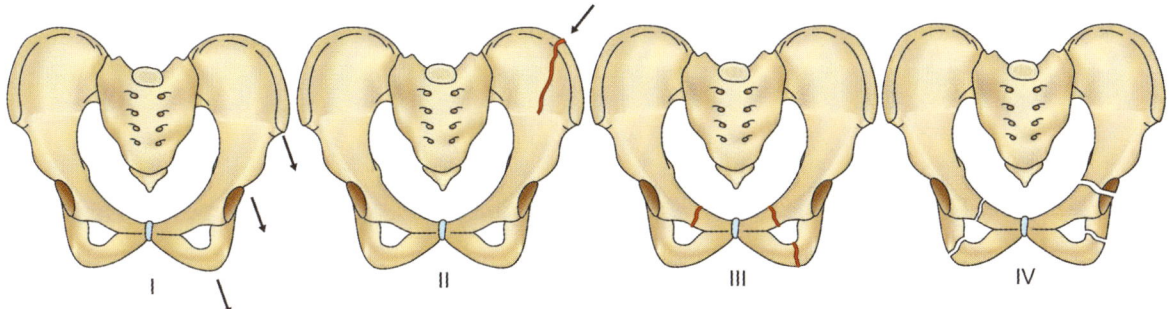

Fig. 4.5: Torode and Zieg classification.

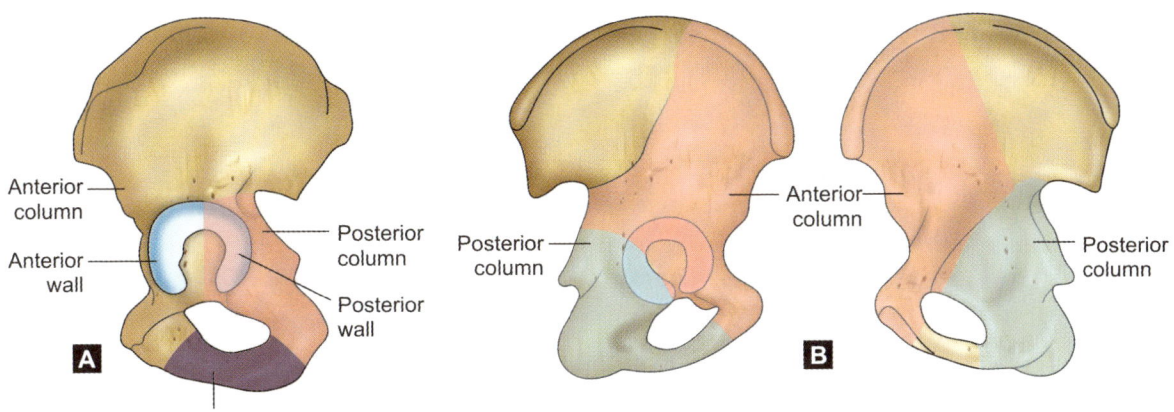

Fig. 4.6a and b: Schematic diagram showing acetabular anatomy and its columns.

On the AP radiograph, there are six basic landmarks (Fig. 4.6c). These are the iliopectineal line, the ilioischial line, the radiographic U or teardrop, the roof of the acetabulum, the anterior rim of the acetabulum, and the posterior rim of the acetabulum. The iliopectineal line is the major landmark of the anterior column. The ilioischial line is formed by the tangency of the X-ray beam to the posterior portion of the quadrilateral surface (internal cortical surface of the acetabulum) and is considered a radiographic landmark of the posterior column.

Obturator oblique view: It is useful to assess the obturator ring, anterior column, and posterior wall. The pelvis is rotated 45° towards the uninjured side with a foam wedge under the affected hip, provides an en face view of the obturator ring, and a profile of the iliac wing (Fig. 4.6d).

Iliac oblique view: It is useful to assess the posterior column and anterior wall. The patient is rolled 45 degrees towards the injured side with a foam wedge under unaffected hip. This provides an en face view of iliac wing and a profile of obturator ring (Fig. 4.6e).

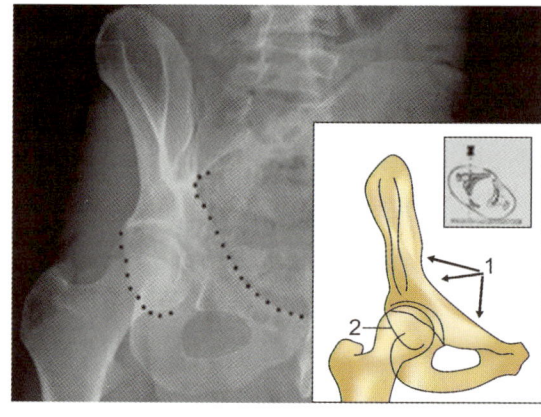

1. Anterior column
2. Posterior wall

Fig. 4.6d: Obturator oblique view.

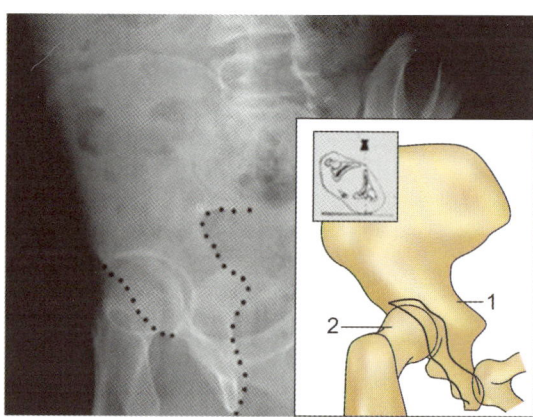

1. Posterior column
2. Anterior wall

Fig. 4.6e: Iliac oblique view.

JUDET AND LETOURNEL (Figs 4.7 to 4.13)

Judet et al. proposed the first systematic classification of acetabular fractures initially published as a thesis by Letournel in 1961. This classification is based on the anatomic pattern of the fracture. It was derived by first understanding the radiograph landmarks on the intact dry innominate and then analysing these landmarks in fracture cases.

Judet and Letournel classification of acetabular fractures is based on the AP view of the pelvis, the obturator (or 45-degree internal, Judet) oblique view, and the iliac (or 45-degree external, Judet) oblique view.

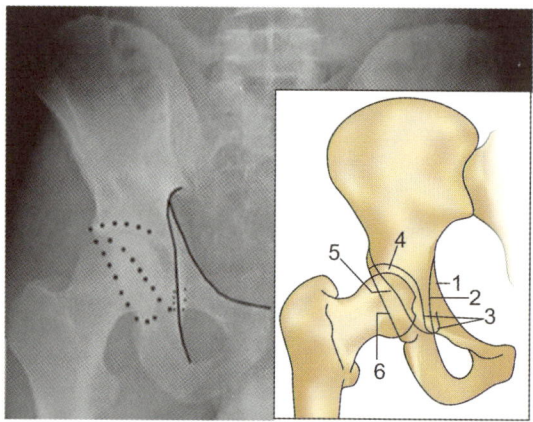

1. Iliopectineal line
2. Ilioischial line
3. Tear drop
4. Acetabular roof
5. Anterior rim of acetabulum
6. Posterior rim of acetabulum

Fig. 4.6c: Anteroposterior view.

This system is an anatomical classification with fractures divided into two groups with five subtypes in each group. The first group, elementary fractures, consists of injuries with one major fracture line. The associated fracture group is also made up of five fracture patterns, each with two or more major fracture lines. The importance of these distinct and separate patterns is well illustrated in the comprehensive text published by Letournel and Judet[14]. They noted that the surgical approach correlates with the fracture classification.

Elementary patterns

1. Posterior wall
2. Posterior column
3. Anterior wall
4. Anterior column
5. Transverse

Associated patterns

1. T-shaped
2. Posterior column and posterior wall
3. Transverse and posterior wall
4. Anterior column with posterior hemi-transverse
5. Both columns

Although several of the associated fracture types involve both columns of the acetabulum, the designation both-column fracture in this classification denotes that none of the articular fracture fragments of the acetabulum maintain bony continuity with the axial skeleton: a fracture line divides the ilium, so the sacroiliac joint is not connected to any articular segment.

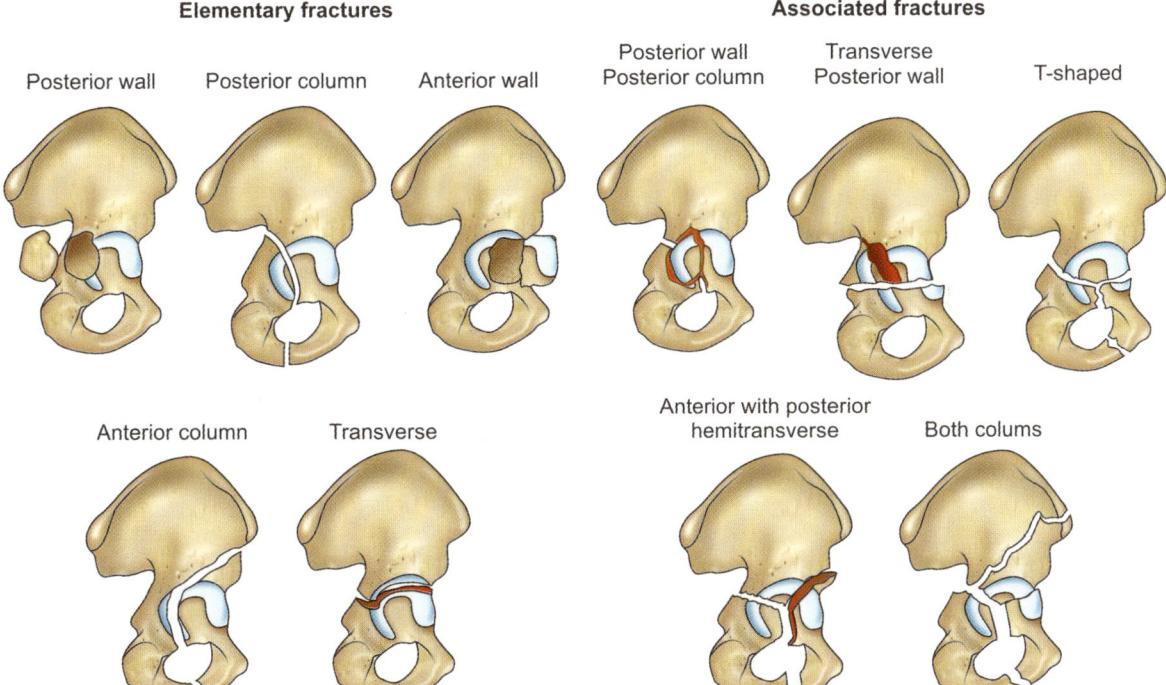

Fig. 4.7: Judet and Letournel classification of acetabulum fracture.

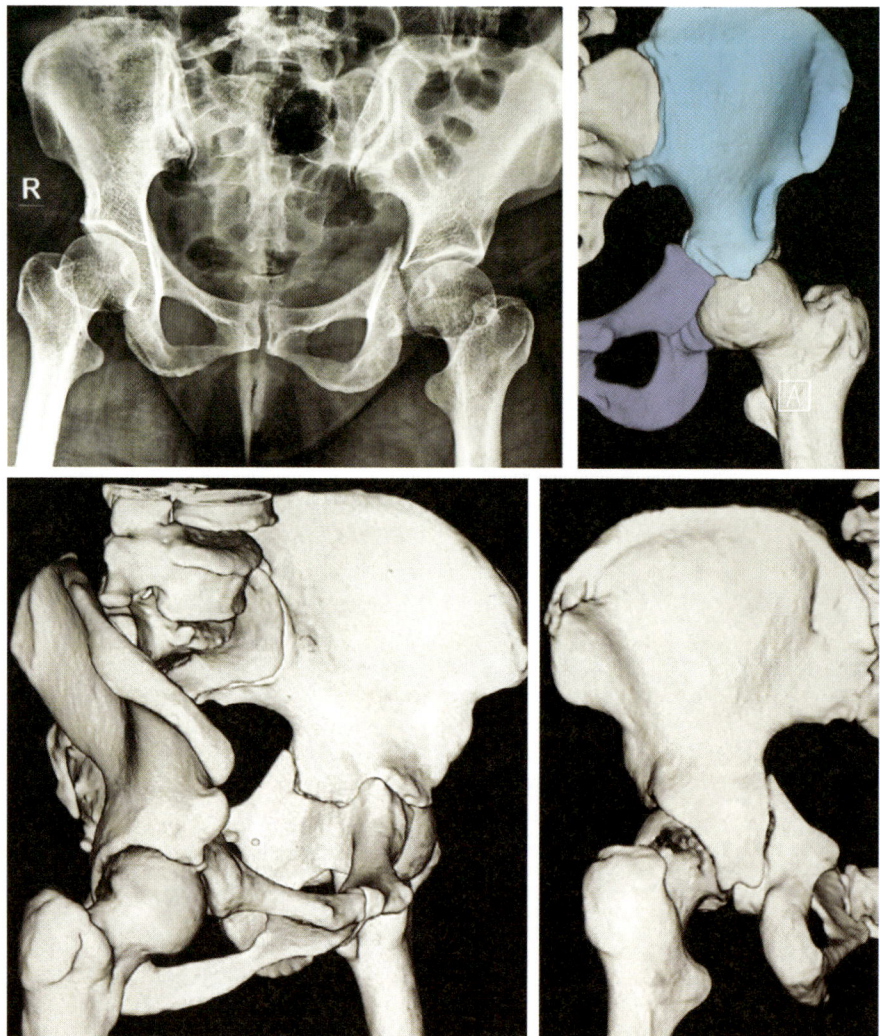

Fig. 4.8: 3D CT scan showing transverse fracture.

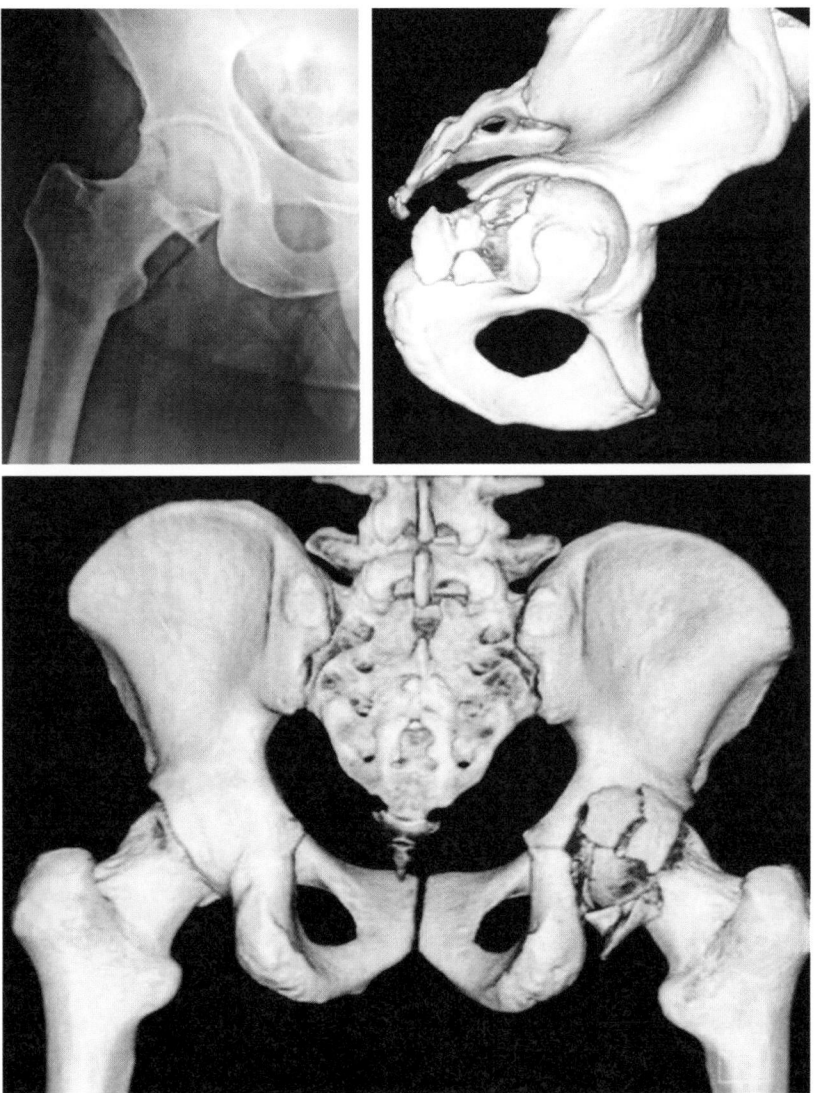

Fig. 4.9: 3D CT scan showing posterior wall fracture.

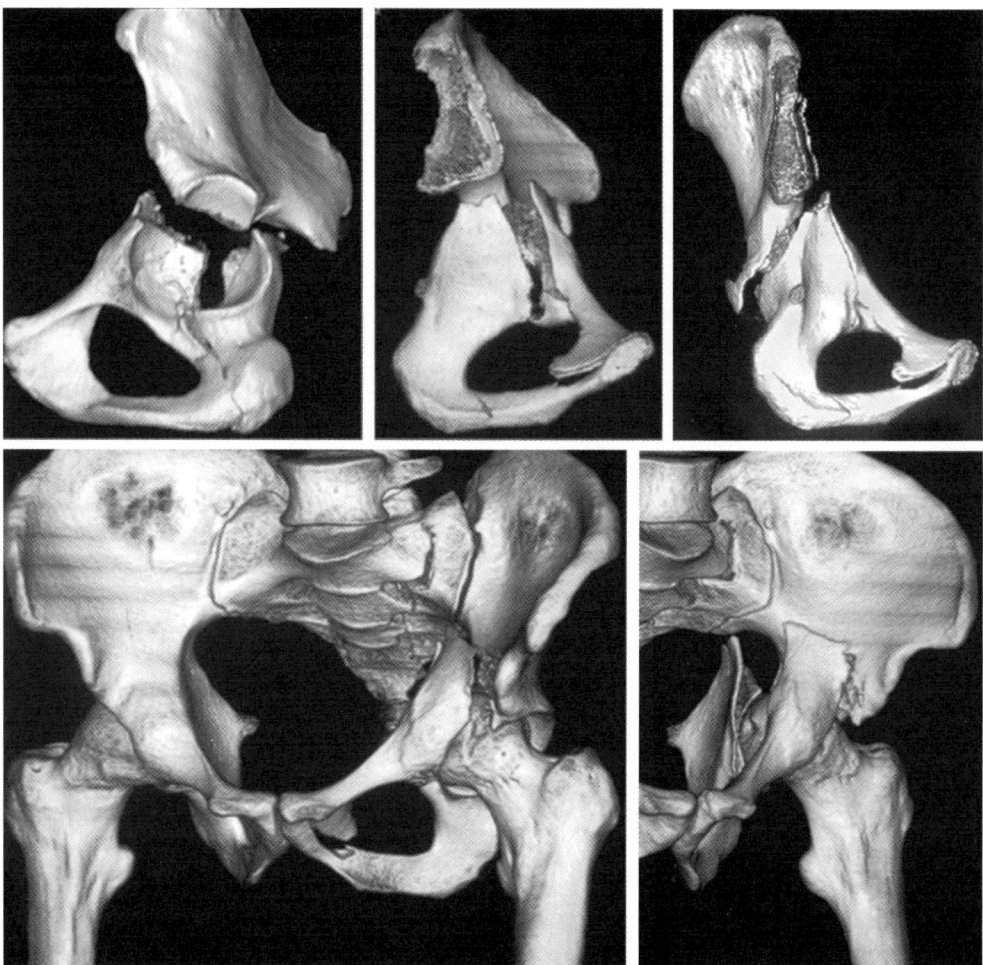

Fig. 4.10: 3D CT scan showing T-type fracture.

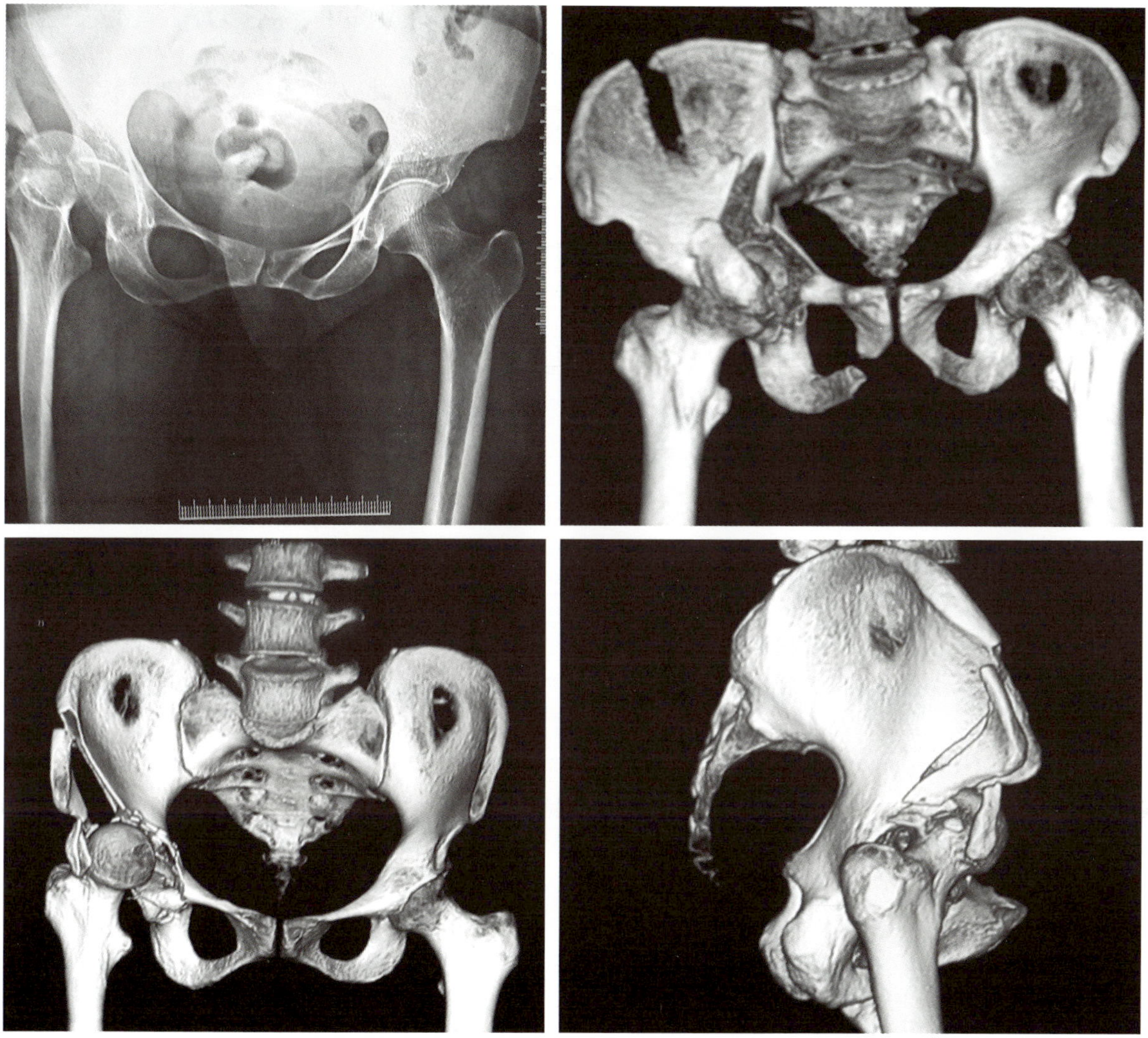

Fig. 4.11: 3D CT scan showing transverse and posterior wall fracture.

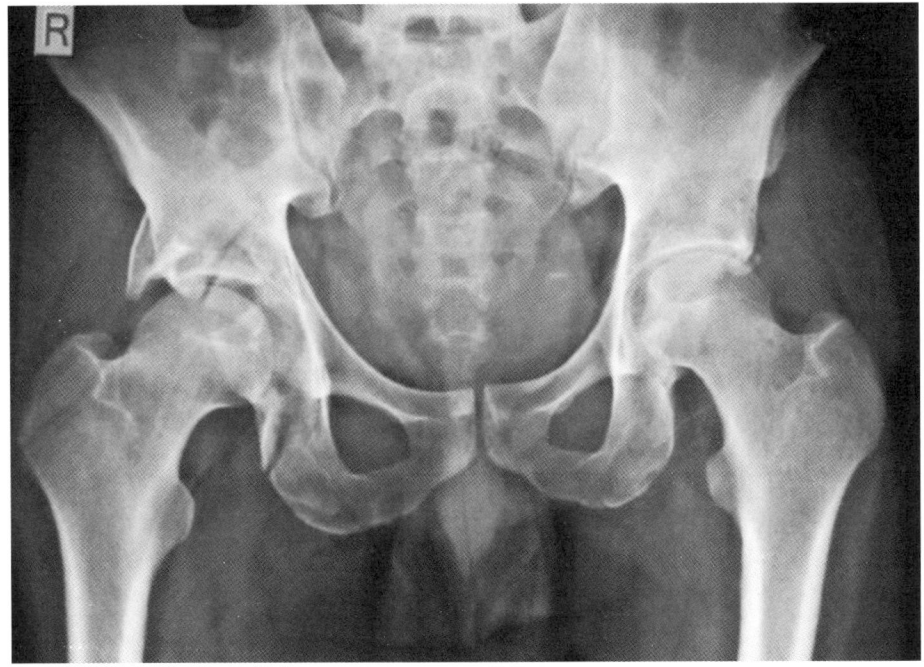

Fig. 4.12: CT scan showing posterior column with posterior wall fracture.

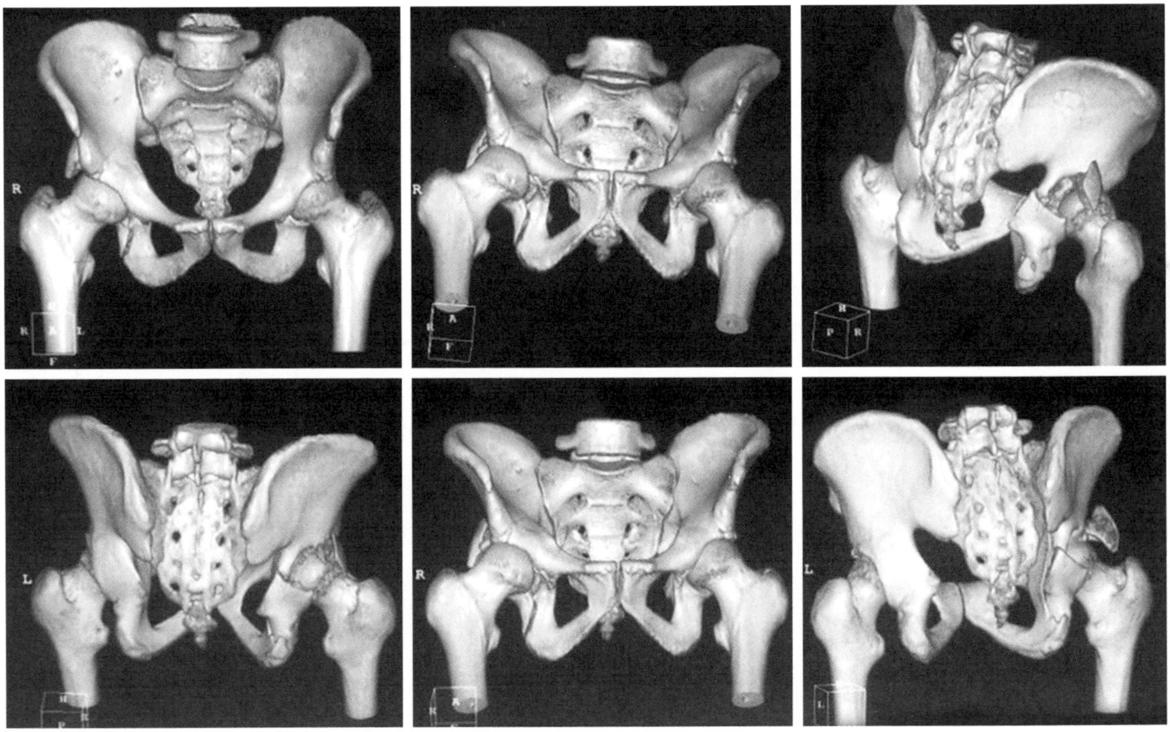

Fig. 4.13: 3D CT scan showing posterior column with wall fracture.

B. AO COMPREHENSIVE CLASSIFICATION OF ACETABULAR FRACTURES (Table 4.1)

TABLE 4.1: AO comprehensive classification

Type A: Partial articular fractures, one column involved
- *A1.* Posterior wall fracture
- *A2.* Posterior column fracture
- *A3.* Anterior wall or anterior column fracture

Type B: Partially articular fractures
- *B1.* Transverse fracture
- *B2.* T-type fracture
- *B3.* Anterior column plus posterior hemitransverse fracture

Type C: Complete articular fracture (both column fracture; floating acetabulum)
- *C1.* Both column fracture, high variety
- *C2.* Both column fracture, low variety
- *C3.* Both column fracture involving sacroiliac joint

3. HIP DISLOCATION

A. EPSTEIN CLASSIFICATION OF ANTERIOR DISLOCATIONS OF THE HIP (Fig. 4.14)

Anterior dislocation are less common and are the result of hyperabduction, external rotation and extension. The degree of hip flexion determined the type of anterior dislocation, with extension leading to a superior pubic dislocation and flexion resulting in an inferior obturator dislocation.

Type I. Superior dislocations, including pubic and subspinous.
- *Type IA.* No associated fractures
- *Type IB.* Associated fracture or impaction of the femoral head
- *Type IC.* Associated fracture of the acetabulum.

Type II. Inferior dislocations, including obturator and perineal
- *Type IIA.* No associated fractures
- *Type IIB.* Associated fractures or impaction of the femoral head/neck
- *Type IIC.* Associated fracture of the acetabulum.

The key to the diagnosis on the plain AP pelvis view is the loss of congruence of the

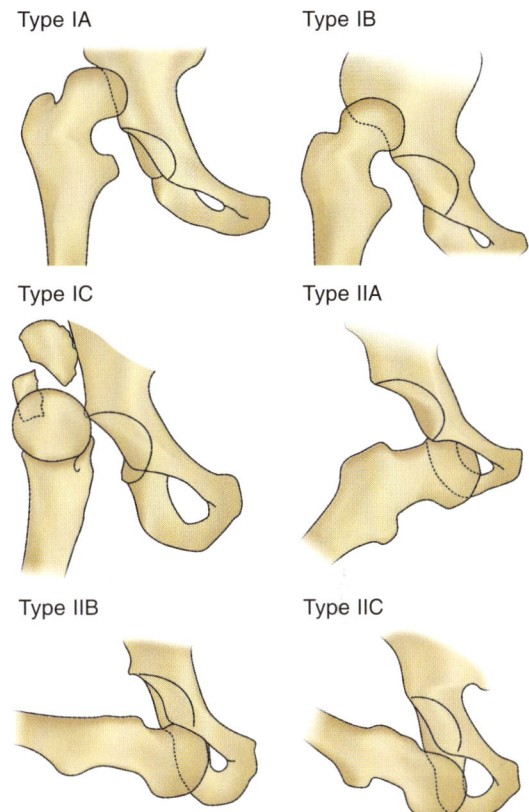

Type IA   Type IB

Type IC   Type IIA

Type IIB   Type IIC

Fig. 4.14: Epstein classification of anterior dislocations of the hip.

femoral head with the roof of the acetabulum. On a true AP view, the head will appear larger than the contralateral head if the dislocation is anterior and smaller if posterior.

B. HIP DISLOCATIONS: POSTERIOR DISLOCATION

Thompson and Epstein Classification of Posterior Dislocations of the Hip (Fig. 4.15)

Type I. Dislocation with or without an insignificant posterior wall fragment.

Type II. Dislocation associated with a single large posterior wall fragment.

Type III. Dislocation with a comminuted posterior wall fragment with or without a large major fragment.

Type IV. Dislocation with fracture of the acetabular floor.

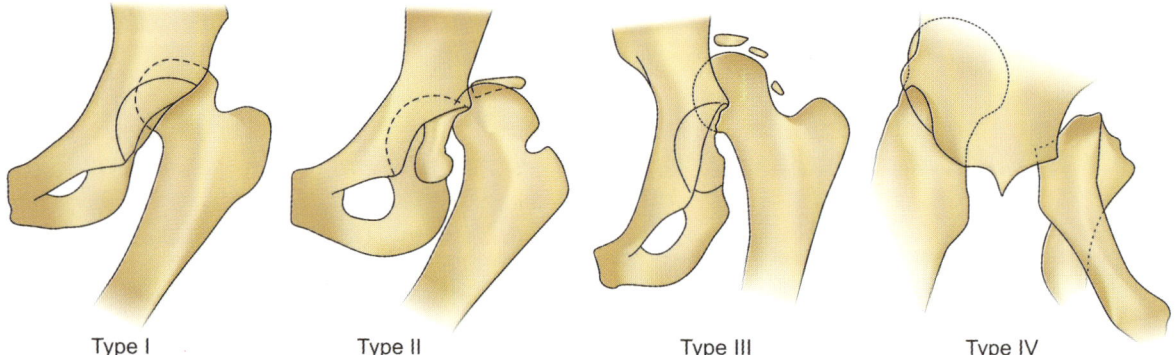

Fig. 4.15: Thompson and Epstein classification of posterior dislocations of the hip.

Type V. Dislocation with fracture of the femoral head.

The position of the hip during axial loading determines the type of injury. Increasing flexion, adduction, and internal rotation (IR) favors pure dislocation, while lesser degrees of each leads to fracture dislocation.

C. PIPKINS CLASSIFICATION

The Thompson and Epstein type V fracture dislocation has been subclassified into four types:

Pipkin Subclassification (Fig. 4.16)

Type I. Posterior hip dislocation with fracture of the femoral head inferior to the fovea centralis.

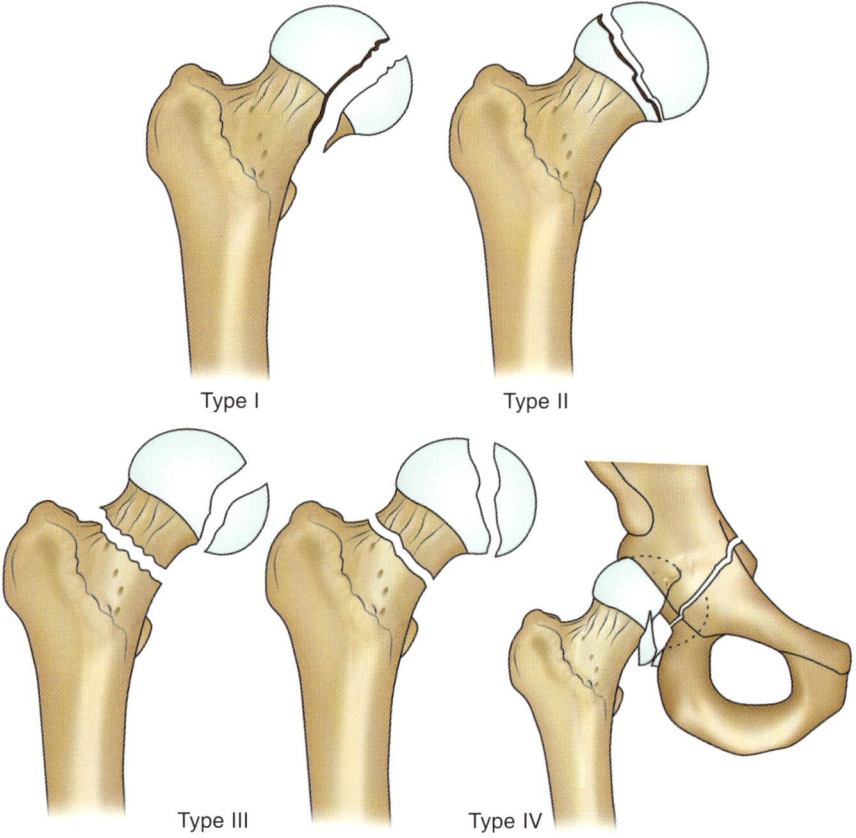

Fig. 4.16: Pipkins classification.

Type II. Posterior hip dislocation with fracture of the femoral head superior to the fovea centralis.

Type III. Type II injury or I associated with fracture of the femoral neck.

Type IV. Types I, II, or III associated with fracture of the acetabular rim.

D. STEWART AND MILFORD CLASSIFICATION

The Stewart and Milford scheme specifically addresses postreduction stability in the case of acetabular fracture, which has prognostic implications (Table 4.2).

TABLE 4.2: Stewart and Milford

Type I	Simple dislocation without fracture
Type II	Dislocation with one or more rim fragments but with sufficient socket to ensure stability after reduction
Type III	Dislocation with fracture of the rim producing gross instability
Type IV	Dislocation with fracture of the head or neck of the femur

E. BRUMBACK CLASSIFICATION

Brumback et al classification can be used for anterior or posterior dislocations . Brumback's classification takes into account the size of the head fragment, the direction of the dislocation, and the stability of the hip (Table 4.3).

4. FEMORAL NECK FRACTURES

Classification by anatomic location
- Subcapital
- Transcervical
- Basocervical

A. PAUWELS CLASSIFICATION (Fig. 4.18)

The Pauwels classification of femoral neck fractures is based on the angle the fracture forms with the horizontal plane. As fracture progresses from type I to type III, the obliquity of the fracture line increases and, theoretically, the shear forces at the fracture site also increase.

Type I—30°

Type II—50°

Type III—70°

B. GARDEN CLASSIFICATION (Fig. 4.19)

The Garden classification is the most commonly used classification system and is based on the degree of displacement on AP X-ray of hip joint by determining the relation of trabecular lines in the femoral head to those in the acetabulum.

TABLE 4.3: Brumback classification of femoral head fractures (Fig. 4.17)

Type 1	Posterior hip dislocation with fracture of the femoral head involving the inferomedial portion of the femoral head
1A	With minimum or no fracture of the acetabular rim and staple hip joint after reduction
1B	With significant acetabular rim and stable joint after reconstruction
Type 2	Posterior hip dislocation with fracture of the femoral head involving the supermedial portion of the femoral head
2A	With minimum or no fracture of the acetabular rim and stable joint after reduction
2B	With significant acetabular fracture and hip joint instability
Type 3	Dislocation of the hip (unspecified direction) with femoral neck fracture
3A	Without fracture of the femoral head
3B	With fracture of the femoral head
Type 4	Anterior dislocation of the femoral head
4A	Indentation type: Depression of the superolateral surface of the femoral head
4B	Transchondral type: Osteocartilaginous shear fracture of the weight-bearing surface of the femoral head
Type 5	Central fracture—dislocation of the hip with femoral head fracture

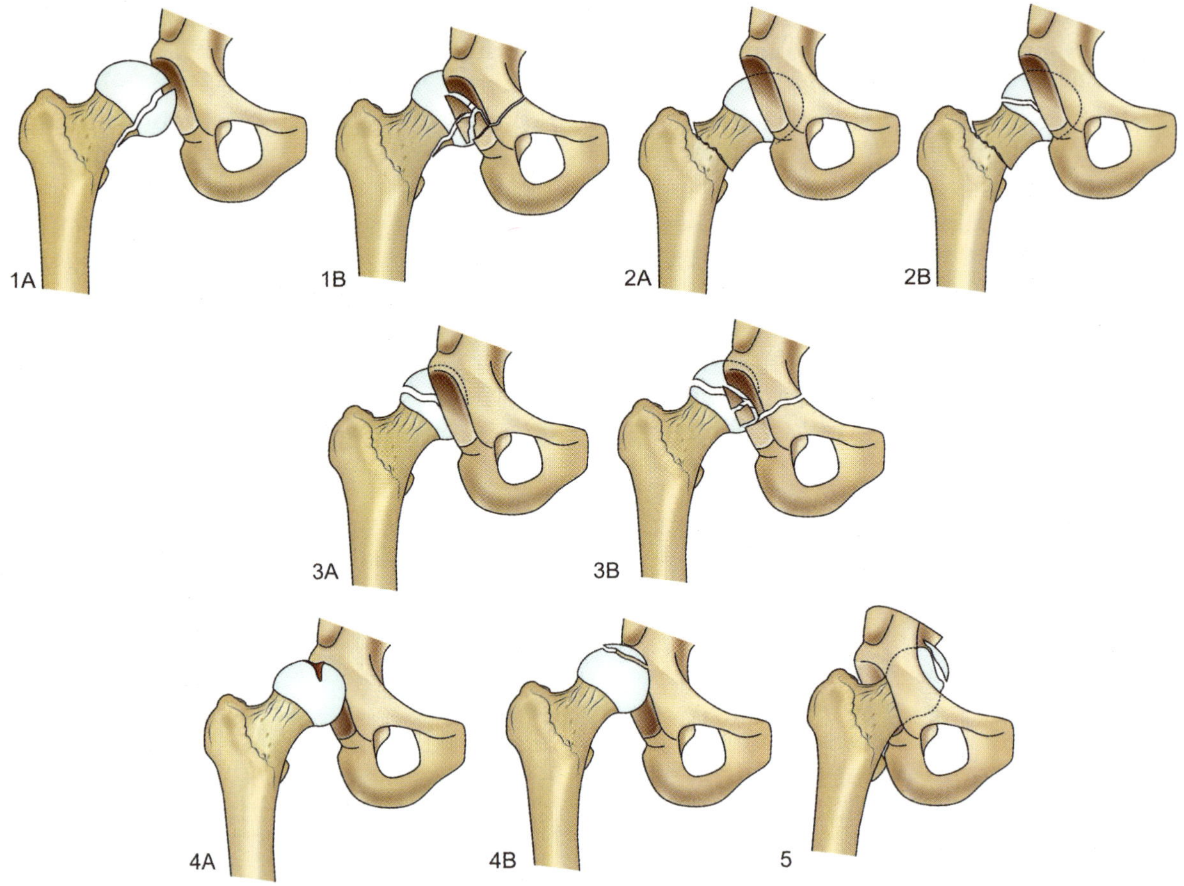

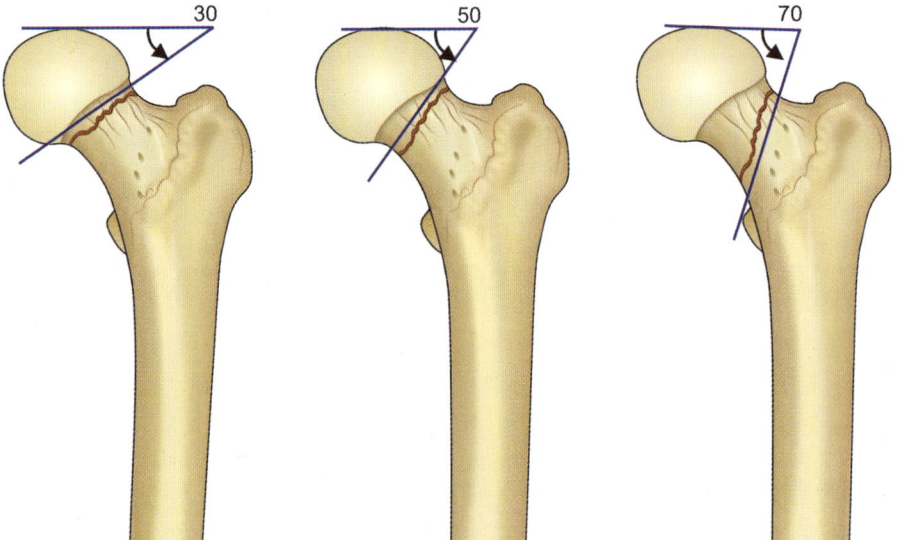

1A   1B   2A   2B

3A   3B

4A   4B   5

Fig. 4.17: Brumback classification of femoral head fractures.

30   50   70

Fig. 4.18: Pauwels' classification.

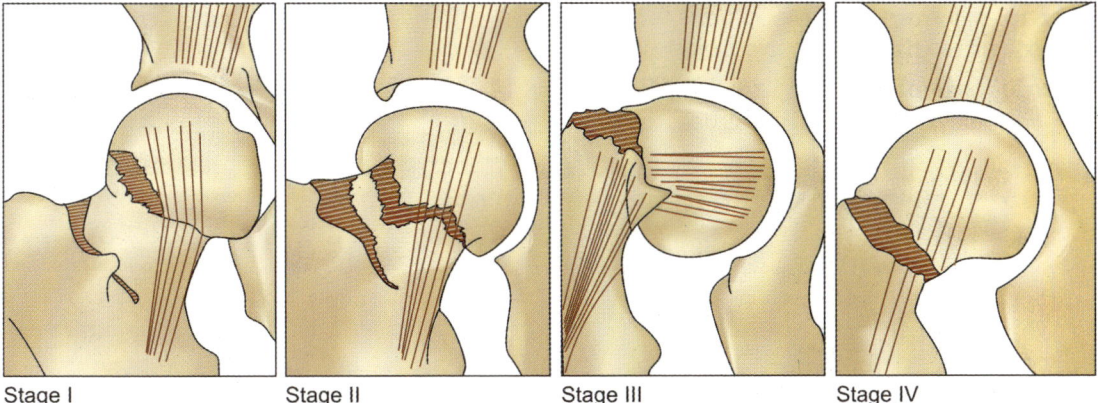

Stage I   Stage II   Stage III   Stage IV

Fig. 4.19: Garden classification.

However, the classification has no role after manipulation or traction application.

The original description, as made on 1961.

Stage I. Incomplete fracture line (valgus impacted)

Stage II. Complete fracture line; nondisplaced

Stage III. Complete fracture line; partially displaced

Stage IV. Complete fracture line; completely displaced.

Stage I
- Incomplete fracture line/valgus impacted.
- Normally aligned trabeculae between acetabulum and head. Trabecular bending in neck with respect to head.

Stage II: Complete nondisplaced fracture with trabecular alignment maintained in all three parts.

Stage III
- Complete with partial displacement.
- Trabecular pattern of the femoral head does not line up with that of the acetabulum and that of head not aligned with neck.
- Head internally rotated and distal fragment externally rotated.
- Some contact is present between head and neck.

Stage IV
- Completely displaced fracture.

- Distal fragment gets further externally rotated and head comes in normal position, so, trabecular pattern of the head assumes a parallel orientation with that of the acetabulum.

5. INTERTROCHANTERIC FRACTURE

A. BOYD AND GRIFFIN CLASSIFICATION (Fig. 4.20)

They were first to mention instability in both coronal and sagittal plane. This classification, included fractures from the extracapsular part of the neck to a point 5 cm distal to the lesser trochanter.

Type I. A single fracture along the intertrochanteric line, stable and easily reducible.

Type II. Major fracture line along the intertrochanteric line with comminution in the coronal plane(posteromedial comminution).

Type III. Fracture at the level of the lesser trochanter with variable comminution and extension into the subtrochanteric region (termed "reverse obliquity" by Wright).

Type IV. Subtrochanteric with intertrochanteric extension with the fracture lying in at least two planes.

Clinical Importance

Type 1. Reduction usually is simple and is maintained with little difficulty. Results generally are satisfactory.

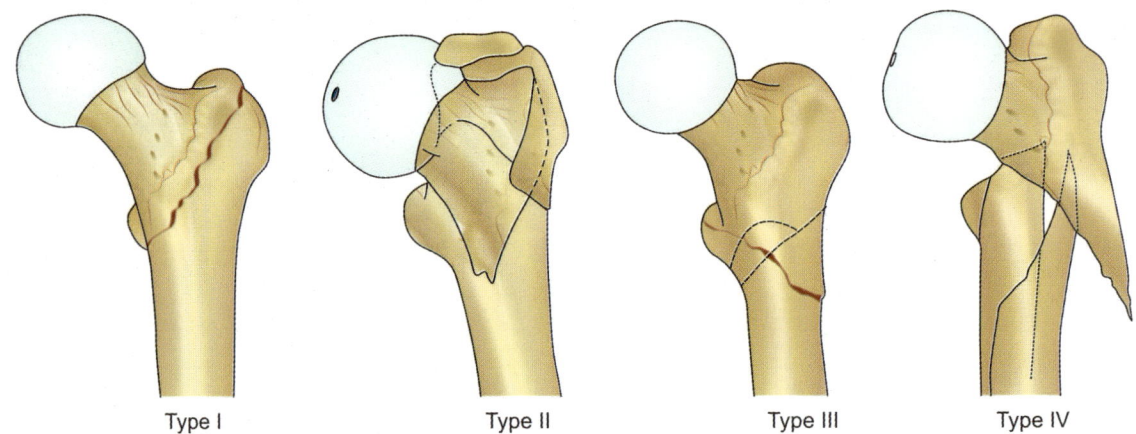

| Type I | Type II | Type III | Type IV |

Fig. 4.20: Boyd and Griffin classification.

Type 2. Reduction of these fractures is more difficult because the comminution can vary from slight to extreme.

Type 3. These fractures usually are more difficult to reduce and result in more complications at operation and during convalescence.

Type 4. If open reduction and internal fixation are used, two-plane fixation is required because of the spiral, oblique, or butterfly fracture of the shaft.

B. EVANS CLASSIFICATION

Type I
Stable
- Undisplaced fractures.
- Displaced but after reduction overlap of the medial cortical buttress make the fracture stable.

Unstable
- Displaced and the medial cortical buttress is not restored by reduction of fracture.
- Displaced and comminuted fractures in which the medial cortical buttress is not restored by reduction of the fracture.

Type II. Reverse obliquity fractures.

According to Evans, posteromedial cortex continuation is important for restoring stability of IT fractures. Based on this he classified IT fractures into Stable and Unstable fractures. Stable fractures have intact or minimally communited posteromedial cortex, while unstable fracture has greater communition of posteromedial cortex. Unstable fractures after reduction can be converted to stable fracture if the posteriomedial cortex opposition can be achieved. Reverse oblique pattern was considered inheritably unstable fracture as distal femur has tendency to drift medially due to adductor pull.

C. JENSEN'S MODIFICATION OF THE EVANS CLASSIFICATION (Table 4.4, Fig. 4.21)

Jansen (1975) later modified Evans classification into three groups.

Displaced or undisplaced stable 2-fragment fractures, unstable 3-fragment fractures with greater or lesser trochanter fracture and 4-fragment fractures.

TABLE 4.4: Evans-Jensen's classification

Type	Description
I	Two-part non-displaced
II	Two-part displaced
III	Three-part fracture without posterolateral support owing to displacement of greater trochanter fragment
IV	Three-part fracture without medial support owing to separate lesser trochanter fragment
V	Four-part fracture without posterolateral and medial support with separate GT and LT fragments

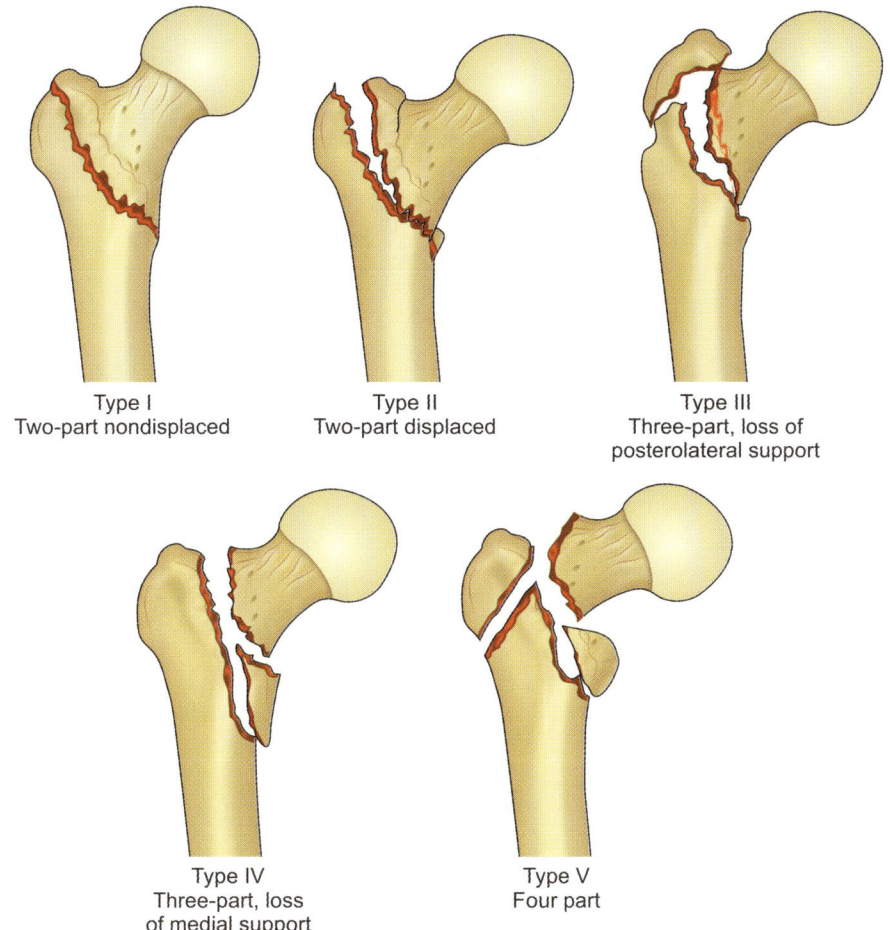

Type I
Two-part nondisplaced

Type II
Two-part displaced

Type III
Three-part, loss of
posterolateral support

Type IV
Three-part, loss
of medial support

Type V
Four part

Fig. 4.21: Jensen's modification of the Evans classification.

D. AO/OTA CLASSIFICATION (Fig. 4.22)

Bone = femur = 3, Segment = proximal = 1, Type = trochanteric = A

A1. Simple (two-part) fractures, with the typical oblique fracture line extending from the greater trochanter to the medial cortex; the lateral cortex of the greater trochanter remains intact.

A2. Fractures are comminuted with a postero-medial fragment; the lateral cortex of the greater trochanter, however, remains intact. Fractures in this group are generally unstable, depending on the size of the medial fragment

A3. Fractures are those in which the fracture line extends across both the medial and lateral cortices; this group includes the reverse obliquity pattern or subtrochanteric extensions.

31-A1. Peritrochanteric simple
- 31-A1.1. Along intertrochanteric line
- 31-A1.2. Through greater trochanter
- 31-A1.3. Below lesser trochanter

31-A2. Peritrochanteric multifragmentary
- 31-A2.1. With one intermediate fragment
- 31-A2.2. With several intermediate fragments
- 31-A2.3. Extending more than 1 cm below lesser trochanter

31-A3. Intertrochanteric
- 31-A3.1. Simple oblique
- 31-A3.2. Simple transverse
- 31-A3.3. Multifragmentary.

Other classification—Gotfried, Kyle, Kulkarni et al.

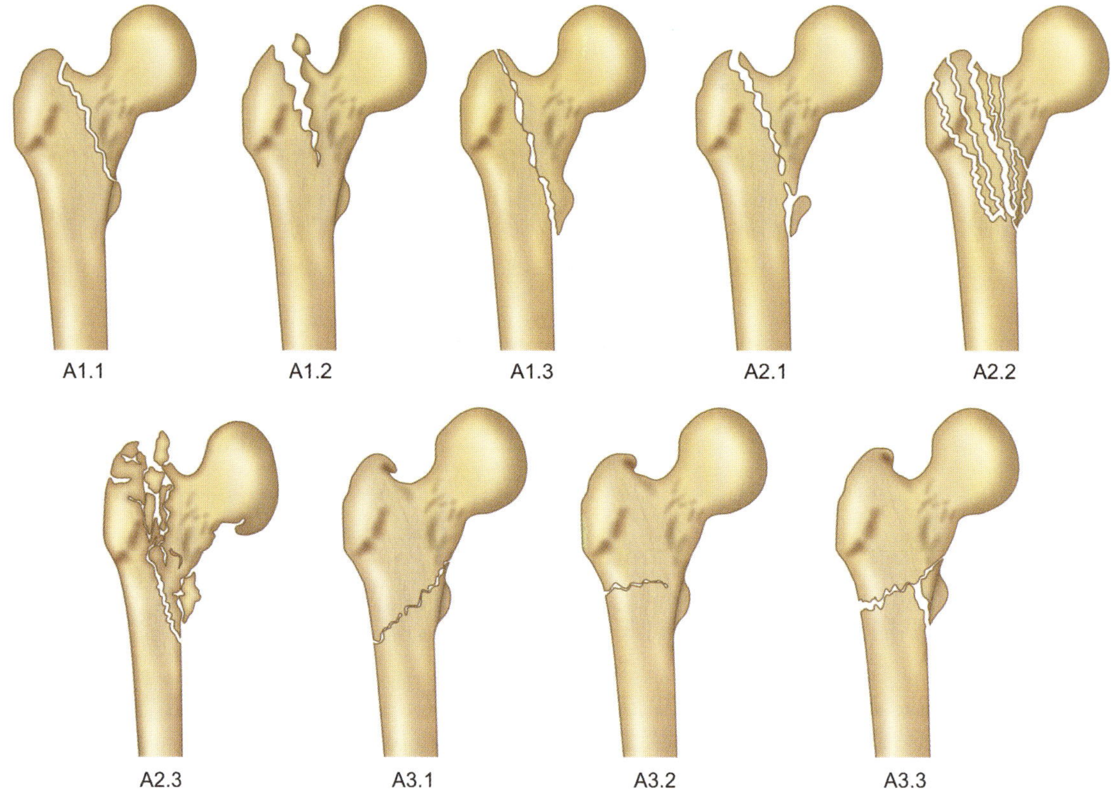

A1.1   A1.2   A1.3   A2.1   A2.2

A2.3   A3.1   A3.2   A3.3

Fig. 4.22: AO/OTA intertrochanteric fracture classification.

6. SUBTROCHANTERIC FRACTURES

A. FIELDING CLASSIFICATION (Fig. 4.23)

Based on the location of the primary fracture line in relation to the lesser trochanter.

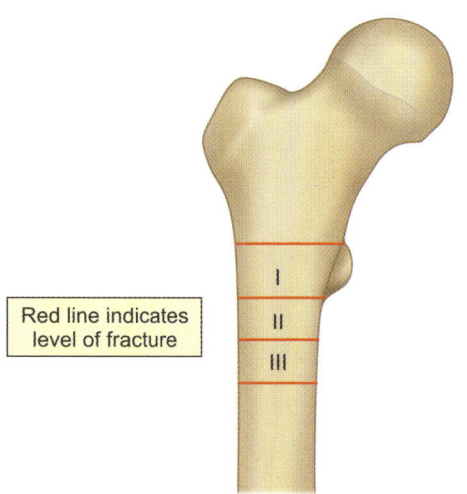

Red line indicates level of fracture

Fig. 4.23: Fielding classification.

Type I. At level of the lesser trochanter

Type II. <2.5 cm below the lesser trochanter

Type III. 2.5 cm to 5 cm below the lesser trochanter.

B. SEINSHEIMER CLASSIFICATION (Fig. 4.24)

The Seinsheimer classification is based on the number of major bone fragments and the location and shape of the fracture lines.

Type I. Nondisplaced fracture or any fracture with <2 mm of displacement of the fracture fragments.

Type II. Two-part fractures.
- *Type IIA.* Two-part transverse femoral fracture.
- *Type IIB.* Two-part spiral fracture with the lesser trochanter attached to the proximal fragment.
- *Type IIC.* Two-part spiral fracture with the lesser trochanter attached to the distal fragment.

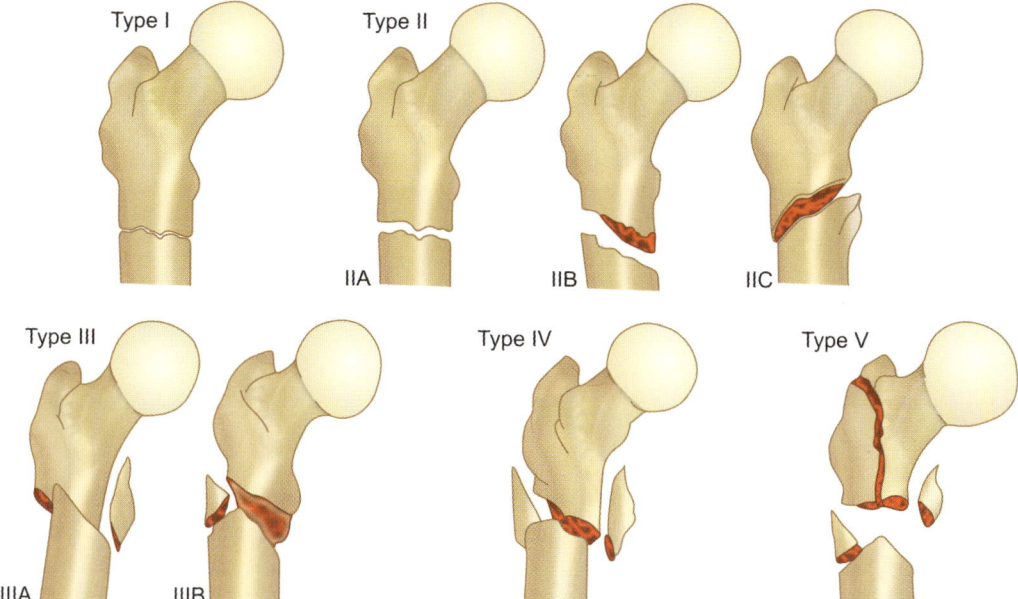

Fig. 4.24: Seinsheimer classification.

Type III. Three-part fractures.

- *Type IIIA.* Three-part spiral fracture in which the lesser trochanter is part of the third fragment, which has an inferior spike of cortex of varying length.
- *Type IIIB.* Three-part spiral fracture of the proximal third of the femur, where the third part is a butterfly fragment.
- *Type IV.* Comminuted fracture with four or more fragments.

- *Type V.* Subtrochanteric-intertrochanteric fracture, including any subtrochanteric fracture with extension through the greater trochanter.

C. RUSSEL–TAYLOR CLASSIFICATION (Fig. 4.25)

It considers the integrity of lesser trochanter and extension of fracture line into pyriformis fossa. It was created in response to development of 1st generation nails and 2nd generation nails (cephalomedullary) as a guide to implant choice.

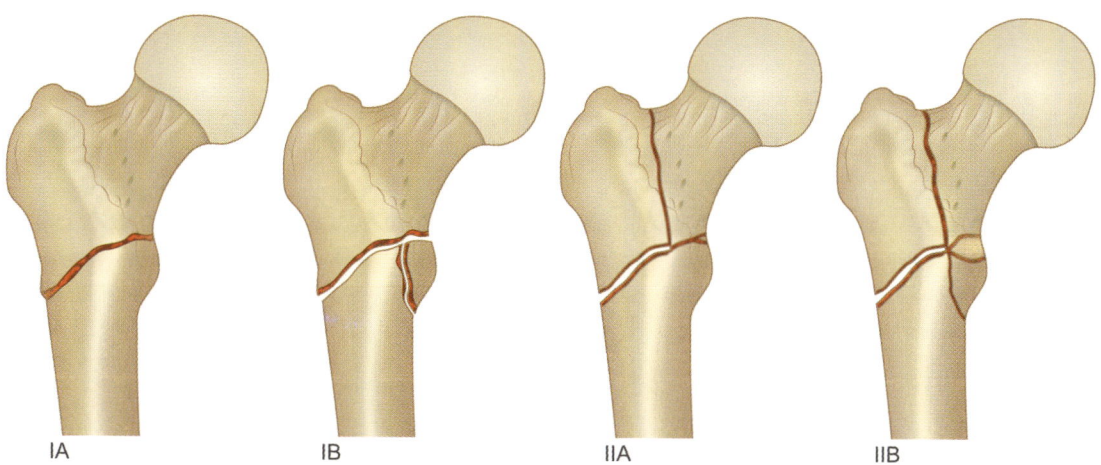

Fig. 4.25: Russel–Taylor classification.

Type I. Fractures do not extend into piriformis fossa:

- Type IA: Lesser trochanter is attached to the proximal fragment.
- Type IB: Lesser trochanter is detached from the proximal fragment.

Type II. Fractures that extend into the piriformis fossa:

- *Type IIA.* No significant comminution or fracture of lesser trochanter
- *Type IIB.* Significant comminution of the medial femoral cortex and loss of continuity of lesser trochanter.

7. FRACTURE SHAFT OF FEMUR

WINQUIST AND HANSEN CLASSIFICATION (Fig. 4.26)

The Winquist and Hansen classification is based on comminution; most useful for determining the need for interlocking nails.

Type 0. No comminution.

Type I. Small butterfly fragment (<25%) or minimally comminuted segment with at least 75% cortical contact remaining between the diaphyseal segments.

Type II. Butterfly fragment or comminuted segment (approx 25–50%) with atleast 50% cortical contact remaining between the diaphyseal segments.

Type III. Large butterfly fragment or comminuted segment (approximately 50–75%) with minimal cortical contact remaining between the diaphyseal segments.

Type IV. Circumferential comminution with no cortical contact at the fracture site/segmentally comminuted.

8. DISTAL FEMUR

It includes both supracondylar cum condylar area.

Supracondylar area is defined as the zone between femoral condyles and the junction of metaphysis with femoral shaft. This comprises approximately the distal 15 cm of the femur, as measured from the articular surface.

AO CLASSIFICATION (Fig. 4.27)

Femur = 3, Distal = 3.

Type A. Extra-articular
- *Type 33-A1.* Simple, two-part supracondylar fracture
- *Type 33-A2.* Metaphyseal wedge
- *Type 33-A3.* Comminuted supracondylar fracture.

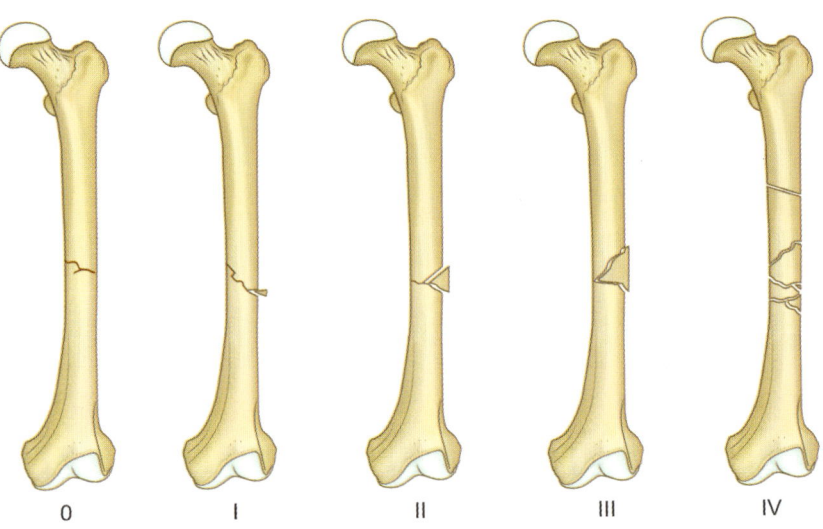

0	I	II	III	IV

Fig. 4.26: Winquist and Hansen classification.

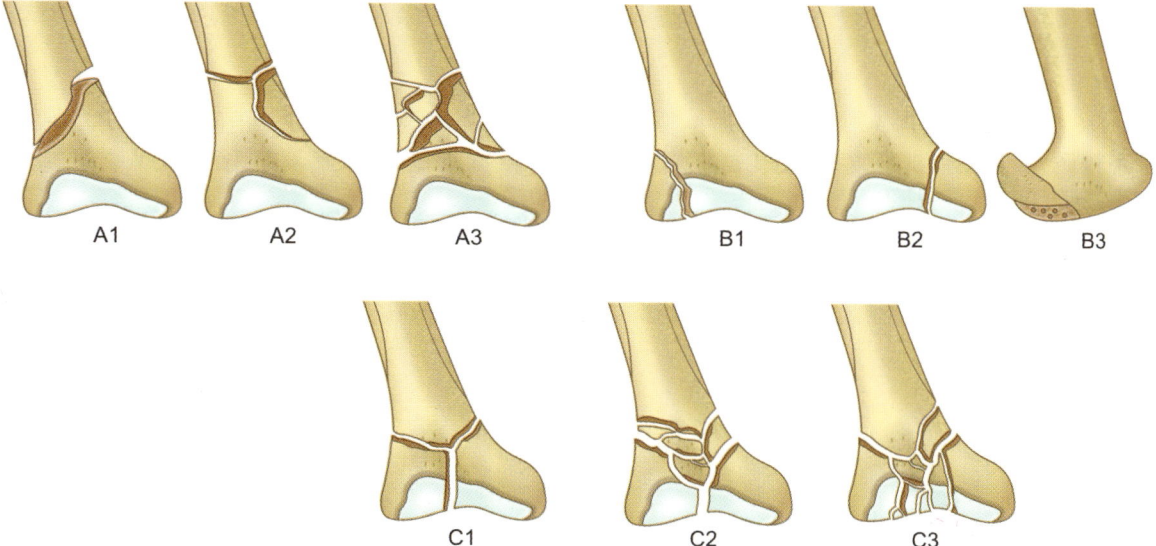

Fig. 4.27: AO/OTA fracture classification of distal femur.

Type B. Unicondylar
- Type 33-B1. Lateral condyle, sagittal
- Type 33-B2: Medial condyle, sagittal
- Type 33-B3: Coronal

Type C. Bicondylar
- *Type 33-C1.* Noncomminuted supracondylar "T" or "Y" fracture.
  Articular simple, metaphyseal simple.
- *Type 33-C2.* Comminuted supracondylar fracture. i.e. articular simple, metaphyseal multifragmentary.
- *Type 33-C3.* Comminuted supracondylar and intercondylar fracture.

9. PATELLAR FRACTURES

It is the largest sesamoid bone of the body having seven articular facets, lateral being the largest and articular cartilage may be as thick as 1 cm.

A. DESCRIPTIVE CLASSIFICATION (Fig. 4.28)

Open versus Closed

Displaced fracture: A displaced fracture of the patella is defined by fracture fragment separation of more than 3 mm or an articular incongruity of 2 mm or more.

Pattern: Stellate, comminuted, transverse, vertical (marginal), polar.

Osteochondral Fracture

Patellar sleeve fracture: In skeletally immature patients in which a distal pole fragment with a large component of the articular surface avulses from the remaining patella.

B. SAUNDERS CLASSIFICATION

Undisplaced
- Stellate
- Transverse
- Vertical

Displaced
Noncomminuted
- Transverse (central)
- Polar (apical or basal)

Comminuted
- Stellate
- Transverse
- Polar
- Highly comminuted.

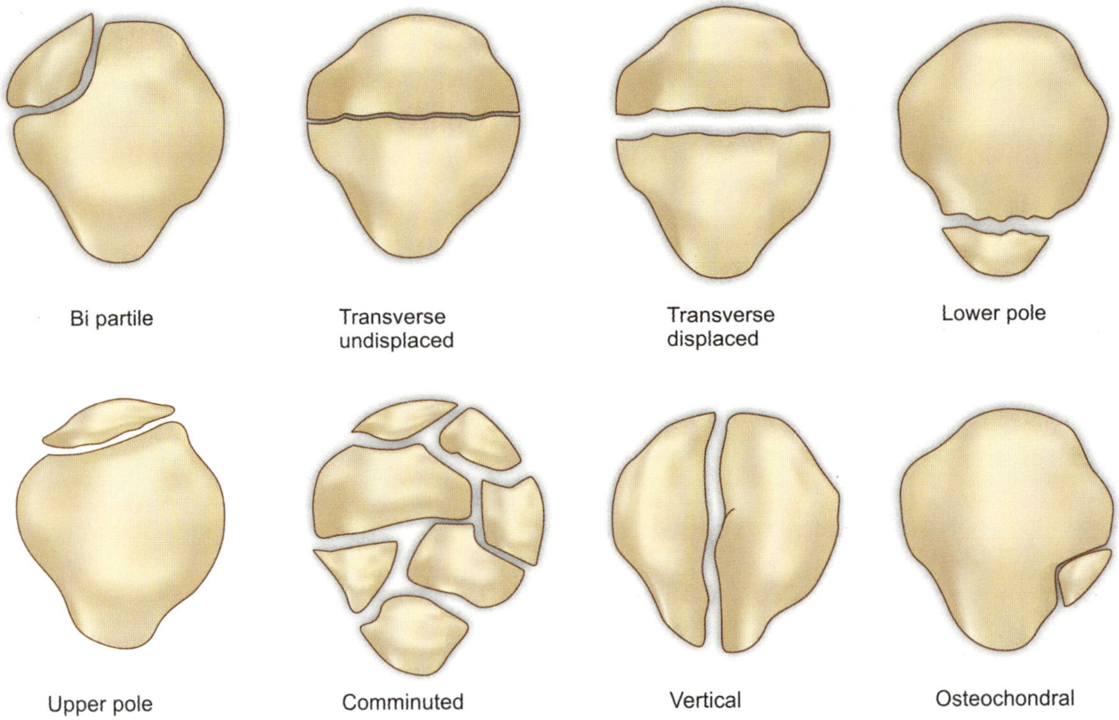

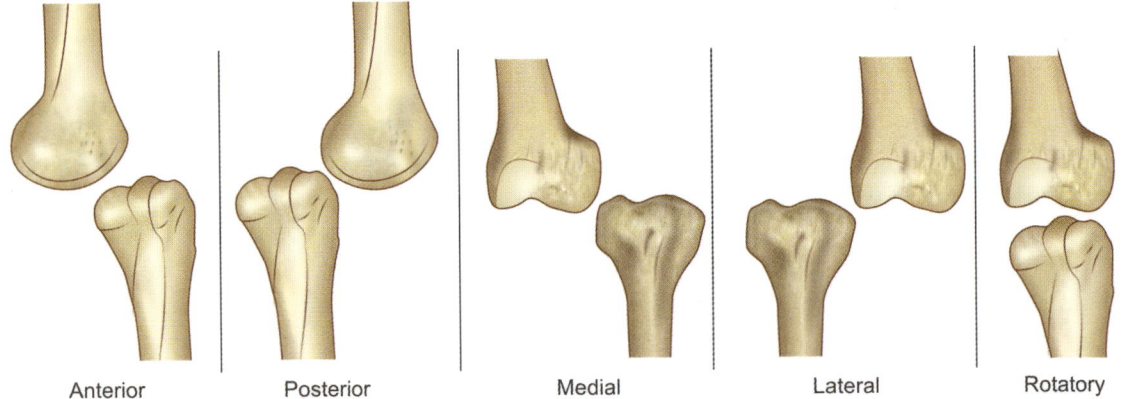

Bi partile

Transverse undisplaced

Transverse displaced

Lower pole

Upper pole

Comminuted

Vertical

Osteochondral

Fig. 4.28: Different types of patella fracture

10. KNEE DISLOCATION

A. DESCRIPTIVE CLASSIFICATION (Fig. 4.29)

The position of the tibia relative to the femur defines the direction of dislocation.

Anterior: Forceful knee hyperextension beyond −30 degrees; most common. Associated with posterior (and possibly anterior) cruciate ligament tear, with increasing incidence of popliteal artery disruption with increasing degree of hyperextension.

Posterior: Posteriorly directed force against proximal tibia of flexed knee; "dashboard" injury. Accompanied by anterior and posterior ligament disruption and popliteal artery compromise with increasing proximal tibia displacement.

Anterior

Posterior

Medial

Lateral

Rotatory

Fig. 4.29: Knee dislocation.

Lateral: Valgus force—medial supporting structures disrupted, often with tears of both cruciate ligaments.

Medial: Varus force—lateral and postero-lateral structures disrupted.

Rotational: Varus/valgus with rotatory component. Usually results in buttonholing of the femoral condyle through the articular capsule.

B. SCHENCK

In 1992 described anatomical classification of knee dislocation paying importance to the ligamentous injury (Table 4.5).

11. PROXIMAL TIBIOFIBULAR JOINT SUBLUXATION

OGDEN CLASSIFICATION

Ogden classified tibiofibular subluxations and dislocations into four types (Fig. 4.30):

Table 4.5: Anatomic of knee dislocation Schenck (1962)

I	Single cruciate + collateral	ACL + collateral
		PCL + collateral
II	ACL/PCL	Collaterals intact
III M	ACL/PCL/MCL	LCL + PLC intact
III L	ACL/PCL/LCL + PLC	MCL intact
IV	ACL/PCL/MCL/LCL + PLC	
V	Fracture dislocation	
C	Arterial injury	
N	Nerve injury	

- Subluxation
- Anterolateral
- Posteromedial and
- Superior dislocations.

Anterolateral dislocations were the most common proximal tibiofibular dislocations in Ogden's series.

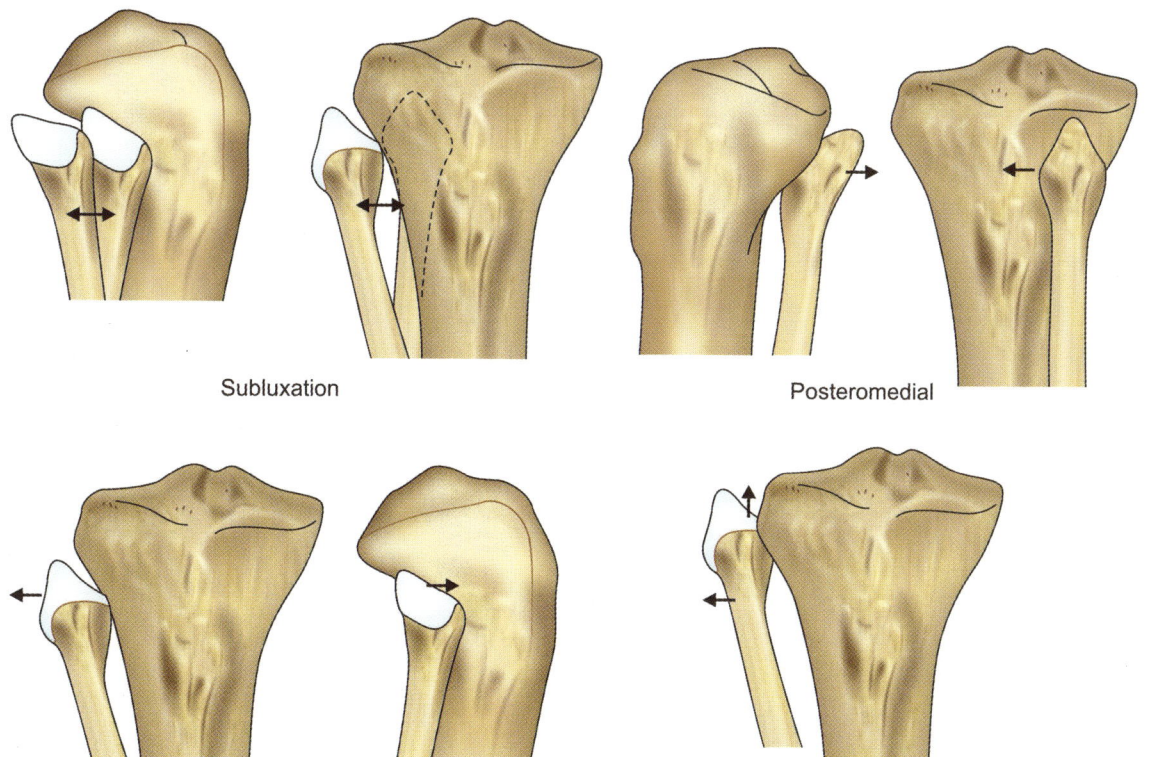

Subluxation   Posteromedial

Fig. 4.30: Ogden classification proximal tibiofibular joint subluxation.

12. TIBIAL PLATEAU FRACTURES

A. SCHATZKER CLASSIFICATION (Fig. 4.31)

Types I-VI. Types I–III are relatively lower energy injury, as compared to types IV–VI.

Type I. Lateral plateau, split fracture.

Common in younger patients without osteoporotic bones. MCL injury is frequent in this type.

Type II. Lateral plateau, split depression fracture.

Most common type. If the depression is more than 5 to 8 mm, or instability is present, most should be treated by open reduction.

Type III. Pure central depression. The articular surface is driven into the plateau. The lateral cortex is intact. Pure depression fracture is rare and occurs in osteoporotic bones.

Type IV. Medial plateau fracture.

The tibial spines often are involved. These fractures tend to angulate into varus.

These fractures had the worst prognosis and more the fracture line moves laterally, more is the risk of associated complications. Chan et al found a high incidence of associated ACL tears in posteromedial fracture patterns.

Type V. Bicondylar plateau fracture.

Both tibial plateaus are split off. The distinguishing feature is that the metaphysis and diaphysis retain continuity.

Type VI. Plateau fracture with metaphyseal–diaphyseal dissociation.

A transverse or oblique fracture of the proximal tibia is present in addition to a fracture of one or both tibial condyles and articular surfaces.

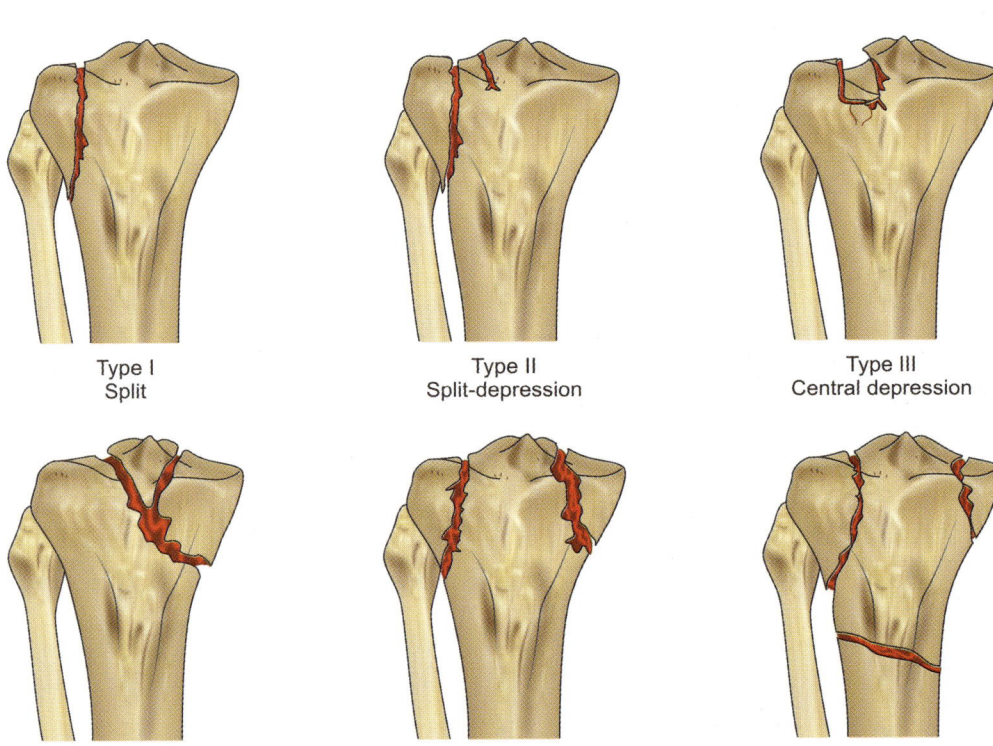

Type I
Split

Type II
Split-depression

Type III
Central depression

Type IV
Split fracture, medial plateau

Type V
Bicondylar fracture

Type VI
Dissociation of metaphysis
and diaphysis

Fig. 4.31: Schatzker classification.

B. HOHL AND MOORE CLASSIFICATION (Fig. 4.32)

The classification distinguishes between five primary fracture patterns and five fracture-dislocation patterns, with fracture-dislocations occurring one seventh as frequently as fractures.

Tibial plateau fracture patterns according to Hohl and Moore include:
- *Type I*—minimally displaced
- *Type II*—local compression
- *Type III*—split compression
- *Type IV*—total condyle
- *Type V*—bicondylar

C. HOHL AND MOORE FRACTURE DISLOCATION CLASSIFICATION (Fig. 4.33)

I. *Coronal split fracture*: The fracture involves the medial side (apparent on lateral view) and has a fracture running at 45° to the medial plateau in an oblique coronal-transverse plane. The fracture may extend to the lateral side, and avulsion fracture of the fibular styloid, insertion of the cruciates, and tubercle of Gerdy are common.

II. *Entire condylar fracture*: This fracture dislocation may involve the medial or lateral plateau and is distinguished from the type IV

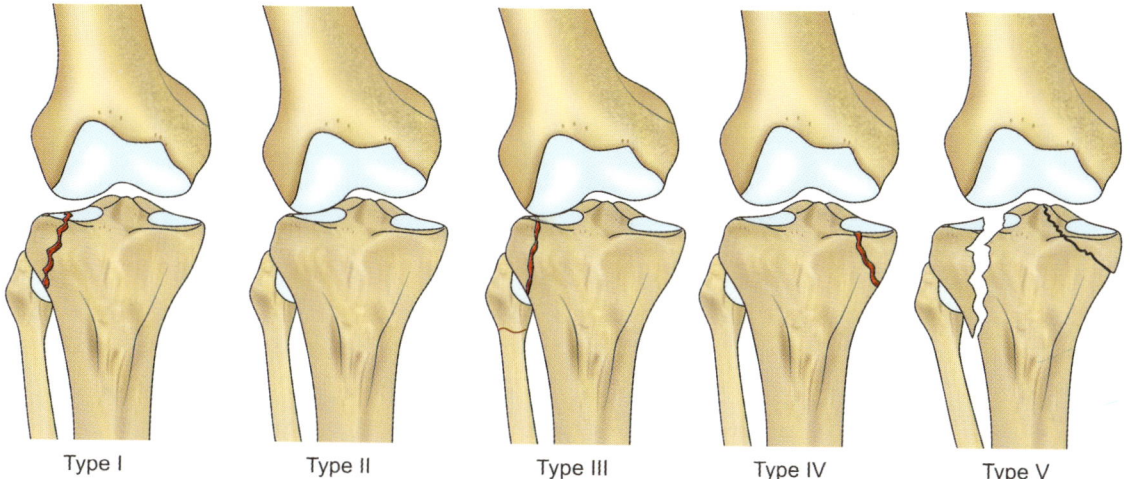

| Type I | Type II | Type III | Type IV | Type V |

Fig. 4.32: Classification of tibial plateau fractures as described by Hohl and Moore.

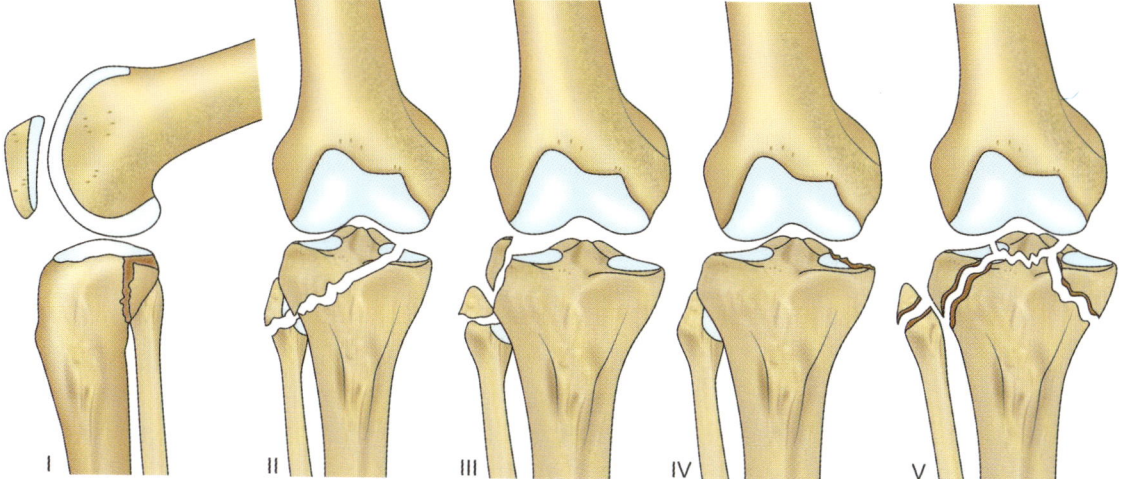

| I | II | III | IV | V |

Fig. 4.33: Hohl and Moore classification of proximal tibial fracture dislocation.

fracture by a fracture line extending into the opposite compartment beneath the inter-condylar eminence. The opposite collateral ligament is involved in half of fractures, resulting in fracture or dislocation of proximal fibula.

III. *Rim avulsion fracture*: Involves almost exclusively the lateral plateau, with avulsion fragment of the capsular attachment, tubercle of Gerdy, or the plateau. Disruption of either or both cruciate ligaments is common. Meniscal injury is rare but neurovascular injury has been reported in approximately 30% cases and nearly all type III fractures are unstable.

IV. *Rim compression fracture*: Almost always unstable. Opposite collateral ligament and usually cruciate ligament are fractured and allow tibia to sublux to the extent that femoral condyle compress a portion of anterior/posterior/middle articular rim.

V. *Four part fracture*: Nealy always unstable. Neurovascular injury is common than the other types. Both collateral ligament complexes are disrupted with the bicondylar fracture and the stabilization provided by the cruciates is lost because the intercondylar eminence is a separate fragment.

13. FLOATING KNEE INJURY

A. LETS et al CLASSIFICATION (Fig. 4.34)

Type A. Both femur and tibia diaphyseal closed fracture.

Type B. Metaphysis (femur/tibia) and diaphysis (tibia/femur) closed fracture.

Type C. Epiphysis (femur/tibia) and diaphysis (tibia/femur).

Type D. One fracture is open with major STI.

Type E. Both fractures are open with major STI.

Their basic recommendation for treatment of these injuries is that at least one fracture (usually the tibial) must be rigidly fixed by internal fixation. Open fractures with major soft tissue injury should be left open and stabilized with external fixation.

B. BOHN AND DURBAN MODIFICATION

Type I. Double shaft fractures, i.e. both femur and tibia shaft fractures.

Type II. One juxta-articular fracture.
- *IIA*: One epiphyseal fracture and one meta-physeal/diaphyseal fracture.

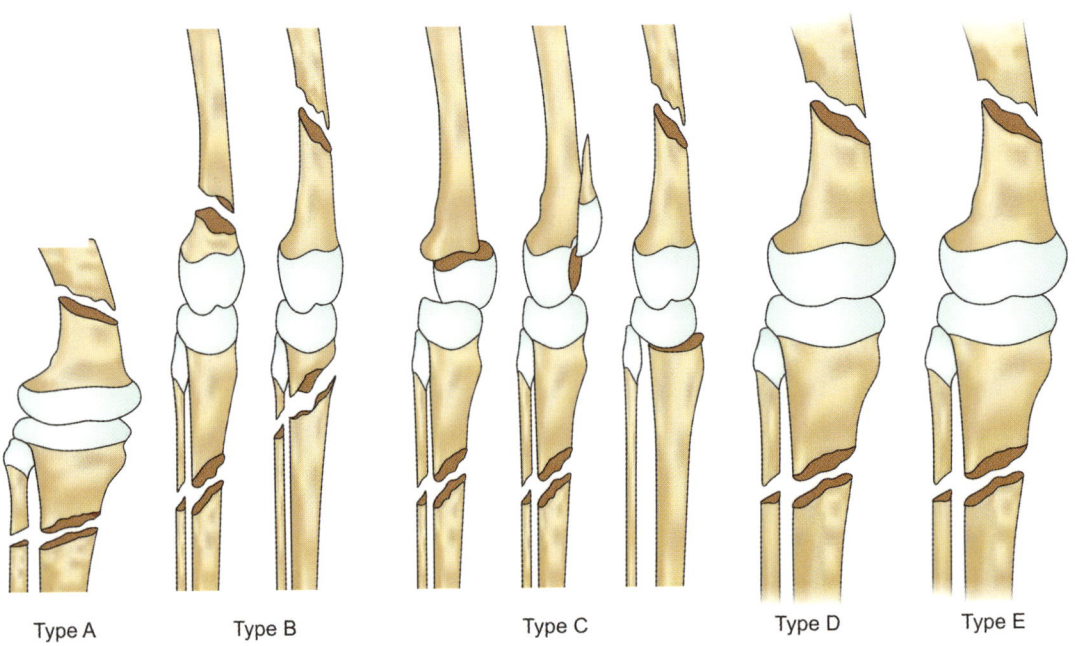

| Type A | Type B | Type C | Type D | Type E |

Fig. 4.34: Lets et al classification of knee dislocation.

- *IIB*: Both epiphyseal fractures (distal femur and proximal tibia)
- *IIC*: Femur and/or tibia fractured at two sites.

C. FRASER CLASSIFICATION (Table 4.6)

TABLE 4.6: Fraser classification (Fig. 4.35)

Types I	Both fractures involve the shaft without articular involvement of the knee
Types II	Articular involvement of the knee
Type IIa	Femoral shaft and tibial plateau fractures
Type IIb	Fractures of the distal femur and the shaft of the tibia
Type IIc	Fractures of the distal femur and tibial plateau

14. TIBIAL/FIBULAR SHAFT

Many classification system has been proposed for fracture shaft of tibia since a long time, but only to be replaced by another.

- Ellis
- Nicoll
- Henley
- Johner and Wruh's
- Trafton

Currently the classification system proposed by AO-OTA group is used most commonly.

A. AO–OTA (Table 4.7)

Tibia/Fibula = 4, Diaphysis = 2.

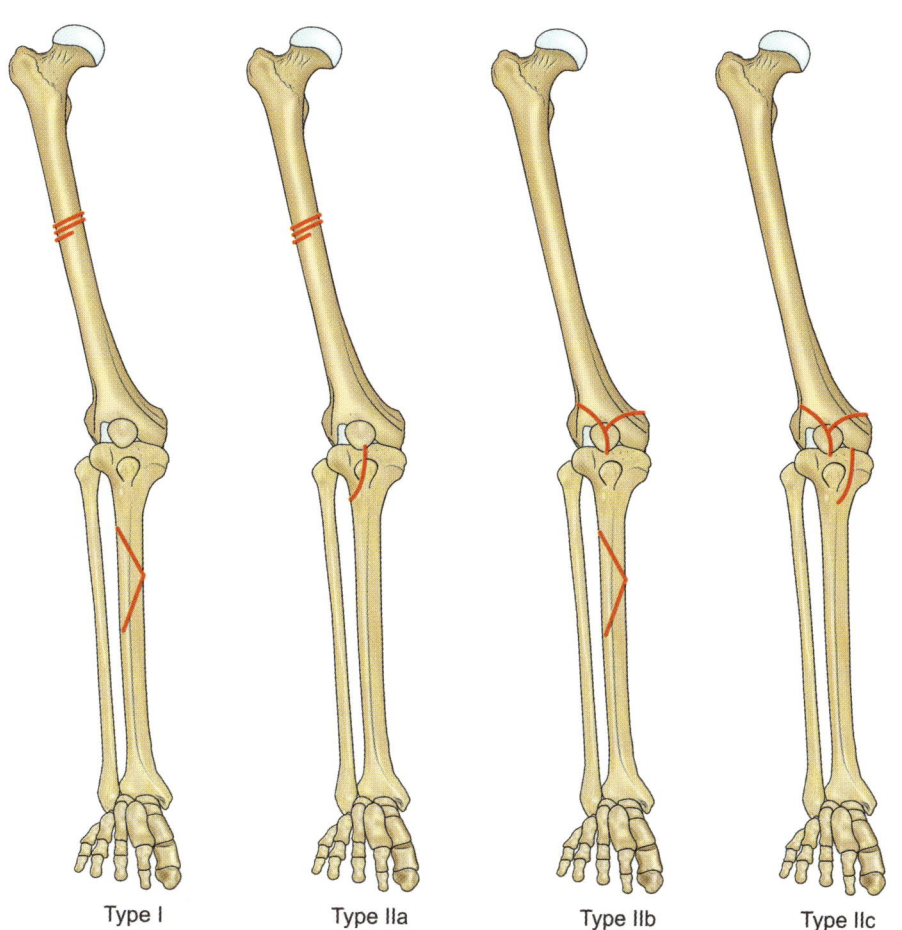

| Type I | Type IIa | Type IIb | Type IIc |

Fig. 4.35: Fraser classification of floating knee.

TABLE 4.7: Orthopaedic trauma association (OTA)–AO classification of tibial diaphyseal fractures

Type A: Unifocal fractures

Group 42-A1		Spiral fractures
Subgroups	A1.1	Intact fibula
	A1.2	Tibia and fibula fractures at different level
	A1.3	Tibia and fibula fractures at same level
Group 42-A2		Oblique fractures (fracture line >30 degrees)
Subgroups	A2.1	Intact fibula
	A2.2	Tibia and fibula fractures at different level
	A2.3	Tibia and fibula fractures at same level
Group 43-A3		Transverse fractures (fracture line <30 degrees)
Subgroups	A3.1	Intact fibula
	A3.2	Tibia and fibula fractures at different level
	A3.3	Tibia and fibula fractures at same level

Type B: Wedge fractures

Group 42-B1		Intact spiral wedge fractures
Subgroups	B1.1	Intact fibula
	B1.2	Tibia and fibula fractures at different level
	B1.3	Tibia and fibula fractures at same level
Group 42-B2		Intact bending wedge fractures
Subgroups	B2.1	Intact fibula
	B2.2	Tibia and fibula fractures at different level
	B2.3	Tibia and fibula fractures at same level
Group 42-B3		Comminuted wedge fractures
Subgroups	B3.1	Intact fibula
	B3.2	Tibia and fibula fractures at different level
	B3.3	Tibia and fibula fractures at same level

Type C: Complex fractures (multifragmentary, segmental, or comminuted fractures)

Group 42-C1		Spiral wedge fractures
Subgroups	C1.1	Two intermediate fragments
	C1.2	Three intermediate fragments
	C1.3	More than three intermediate fragments
Group 42-C2		Segmental fractures
Subgroups	C2.1	One segmental fragment
	C2.2	Segmental fragment and additional wedge fragment
	C2.3	Two segmental fragments
Group 42-C3		Comminuted fractures
Subgroups	C3.1	Two or three intermediate fragments
	C3.2	Limited comminution (<4 cm)
	C3.3	Extensive comminution (>4 cm)

B. GUSTILO AND ANDERSON CLASSIFICATION OF ALL OPEN FRACTURES

The score should be applied post-debridement and the score may change with each debridement.

Type I
- Wound less than 1 cm long
- Moderately clean puncture, where spike of bone has pierced the skin
- Little soft tissue damage
- No crushing
- Fracture usually simple transverse or oblique with little comminution

Type II
- Laceration more than 1 cm long
- No extensive soft tissue damage, flap or contusion
- Slight to moderate crushing injury
- Moderate comminution
- Moderate contamination

Type III
- Extensive damage to soft tissues
- High degree of contamination
- Fracture caused by high velocity trauma

IIIA: Adequate soft tissue cover
- >10 cm, high energy
- Adequate tissue for coverage
- Includes segmental or extensively comminuted fractures or bone loss even if wound <10 cm
- Gunshot wound

IIIB: Inadequate soft tissue cover, periosteal stripping and bone exposure, massive contamination. A local or free flap is required

IIIC: Any fracture with an arterial injury which requires repair.

15. PILON FRACTURE

All fractures of the distal tibia involving the distal articular surface should be classified as pilon fractures, except medial, lateral and trimalleolar fractures where the posterior malleolus is <1/3rd of the articular surface.

If isolated fracture of the posterior malleolus is more than >1/3rd of the articular surface, than it should be classified as pilon fracture.

A. RUEDI–ALLGOWER CLASSIFICATION (Fig. 4.36)

Type I. No significant articular incongruity; cleavage fractures without displacement of bony fragments.

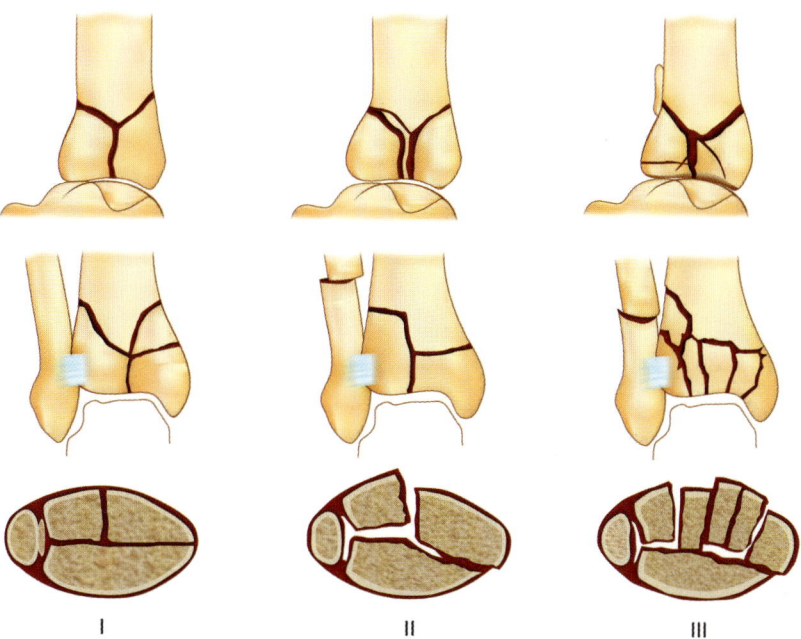

I   II   III

Fig. 4.36: Ruedi–Allgower classification.

Type II. Significant articular incongruity with minimal impaction or comminution.

Type III. Significant articular comminution with metaphyseal impaction.

B. AO–OTA CLASSIFICATION (43) (Fig. 4.37)

Type A. Distal tibial metaphyseal injuries without intra-articular extension.

- *A1*: Simple
- *A2*: Comminuted
- *A3*: Severely comminuted

Type B. Partial articular fractures

- *B1*: Pure split
- *B2*: Split with depression
- *B3*: Depression with multiple fragments

Type C: Fracture involves the entire joint surface

- *C1*: Simple split in the articular surface and the metaphysis
- *C2*: Articular split that is simple with a metaphysis split that is multifragmentary
- *C3*: Fracture with multiple fragments of the articular surface and the metaphysic.

16. ANKLE FRACTURE

A. POTT'S CLASSIFICATION

Pott' first provided the known detailed description of ankle fractures prior to the discovery of medical radiographs. Fractures can be described as unimalleolar, bimalleolar and trimalleolar based on the combined fractures of the lateral, medial and posterior malleoli.

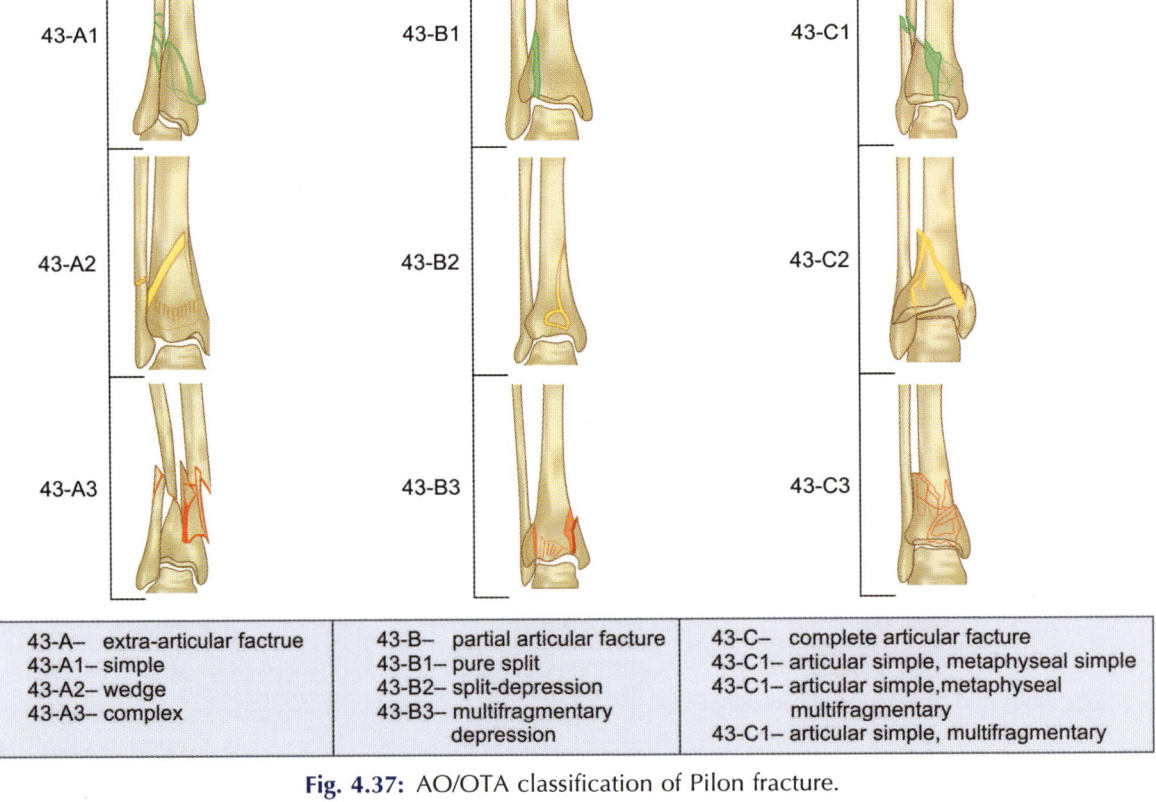

43-A— extra-articular factrue	43-B— partial articular facture	43-C— complete articular facture
43-A1– simple	43-B1– pure split	43-C1– articular simple, metaphyseal simple
43-A2– wedge	43-B2– split-depression	43-C1– articular simple,metaphyseal multifragmentary
43-A3– complex	43-B3– multifragmentary depression	43-C1– articular simple, multifragmentary

Fig. 4.37: AO/OTA classification of Pilon fracture.

Acronyms

- ***Pott's fracture:*** Bimalleoli fracture
- ***Cottons fracture:*** Trimalleoli fracture.
- ***Volkman's fracture:*** Posterior malleolus fracture.
- ***Maisonneuve fracture:*** The fracture of proximal fibula associated with a medial malleolus fracture or deltoid ligament injury.

B. DANIS AND WEBER CLASSIFICATION (Fig. 4.38)

Fractures are categorized into A, B, and C based on the level of the fibular fracture.

Type A. Fractures are below the level of the distal tibial fibular syndesmosis,

Type B. Fractures are at the level of the syndesmosis, and

Type C. Fractures are above the syndesmosis.

C. AO/OTA CLASSIFICATION

The current AO/OTA classification is an extension of the Weber classification. It uses an alphanumeric code, i.e. **44** to provide a detailed morphologic description of rotational ankle fractures. It has three types, nine groups, and **27** subgroups. The three types, A, B, and C, have remained the same as those described in the previous classification.

Type A. Fibula fracture below the syndesmosis
- *Type A1:* Isolated
- *Type A2:* With fracture of medial malleolus
- *Type A3:* With posteromedial fracture

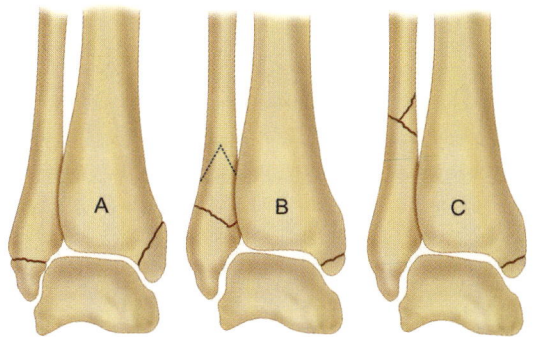

Fig. 4.38: Danis and Weber classification.

Type B. Fibula fracture at the level of syndesmosis
- *Type B1:* Isolated
- *Type B2:* With medial lesion (malleolus or ligament)
- *Type B3:* With medial lesion and fracture of posterolateral tibia

Type C. Fibula fracture above syndesmosis
- *Type C1:* Diaphyseal fracture of the fibula, simple
- *Type C2:* Diaphyseal fracture of the fibula, complex
- *Type C3:* Proximal fracture of fibula.

D. LAUGE–HANSEN CLASSIFICATION

- It employs two words and a number. The first word describes the position of the foot at the time of injury (supination/pronation) and second word, the direction of the deforming force (abduction/adduction/external rotation/internal rotation).
- Four patterns, based on "pure" injury sequences, each subdivided into stages of increasing severity.

1. Supination–external rotation (SER) (Fig. 4.39)—most common mechanism.
- *Stage I:* Disruption of the anterior tibiofibular ligament with or without an associated avulsion fracture at its tibial or fibular attachment.
- *Stage II:* Spiral fracture of the distal fibula at the level of syndesmosis, which runs from anteroinferior to posterosuperior. Ankle remains stable. Its equivalent to Denis-Weber type B.
- *Stage III:* Disruption of the posterior tibiofibular ligament or a fracture of the posterior malleolus.
- *Stage IV:* Transverse avulsion-type fracture of the medial malleolus or a rupture of the deltoid ligament. Ankle becomes unstable.

2. Supination–adduction (SA) (Fig. 4.39)
- *Stage I:* Transverse avulsion-type fracture of the fibula distal to the level of the joint or a rupture of the lateral collateral

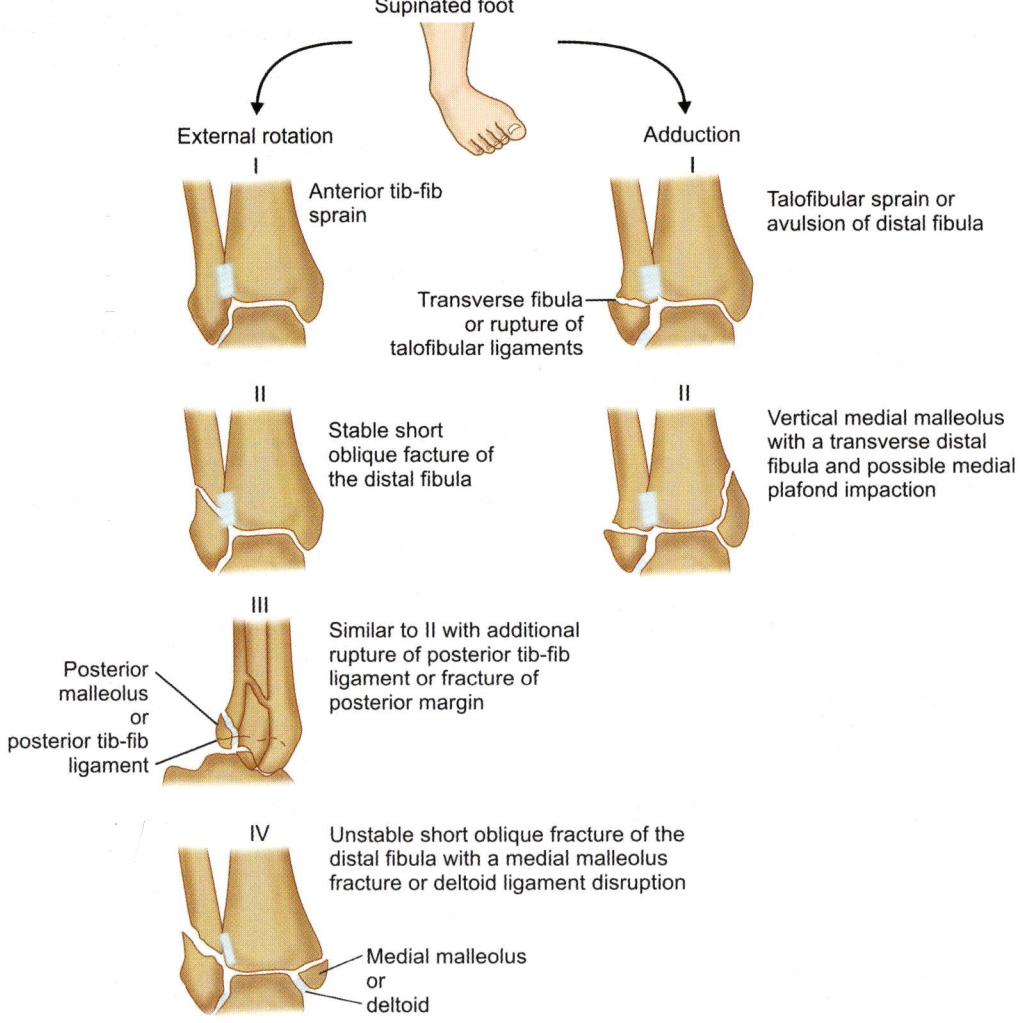

Supinated foot

External rotation

I
Anterior tib-fib sprain

Transverse fibula or rupture of talofibular ligaments

II
Stable short oblique facture of the distal fibula

III
Posterior malleolus or posterior tib-fib ligament

Similar to II with additional rupture of posterior tib-fib ligament or fracture of posterior margin

IV
Unstable short oblique fracture of the distal fibula with a medial malleolus fracture or deltoid ligament disruption

Medial malleolus or deltoid

Adduction

I
Talofibular sprain or avulsion of distal fibula

II
Vertical medial malleolus with a transverse distal fibula and possible medial plafond impaction

Fig. 4.39: The SER mechanism has four stages and SAD mechanism has two stages.

ligaments/talofibular ligament. It is equivalent to Denis-Weber type A.

- *Stage II*: Vertical fracture of medial malleolus. The medial plafond may suffer impaction from the talus and radiographs should be scrutinised carefully for this additional injury. In contradistinction to the other patterns of ankle fracture, surgical stabilisation of SAD2 fracture begins with the initial exposure of the medial malleolus.

3. *Pronation–abduction (PAB)* (Fig. 4.40)
- *Stage I*: Transverse avulsion fracture of the medial malleolus or a rupture of the deltoid ligament.

- *Stage II*: Rupture of the syndesmotic ligaments/anterior tibiofibular ligament or an avulsion fracture at their insertions/chaput fracture.
- *Stage III*: Comminuted fracture of the distal fibula at or above the level of the syndesmosis. (It differs from SER fracture that, lag screw fixation is not possible in this type of fracture and has to be fixed with bridge plating or IMN).

4. *Pronation–external rotation (PER)* (Fig. 4.40)
- *Stage I*: Transverse fracture of the medial malleolus or a rupture of the deltoid ligament.

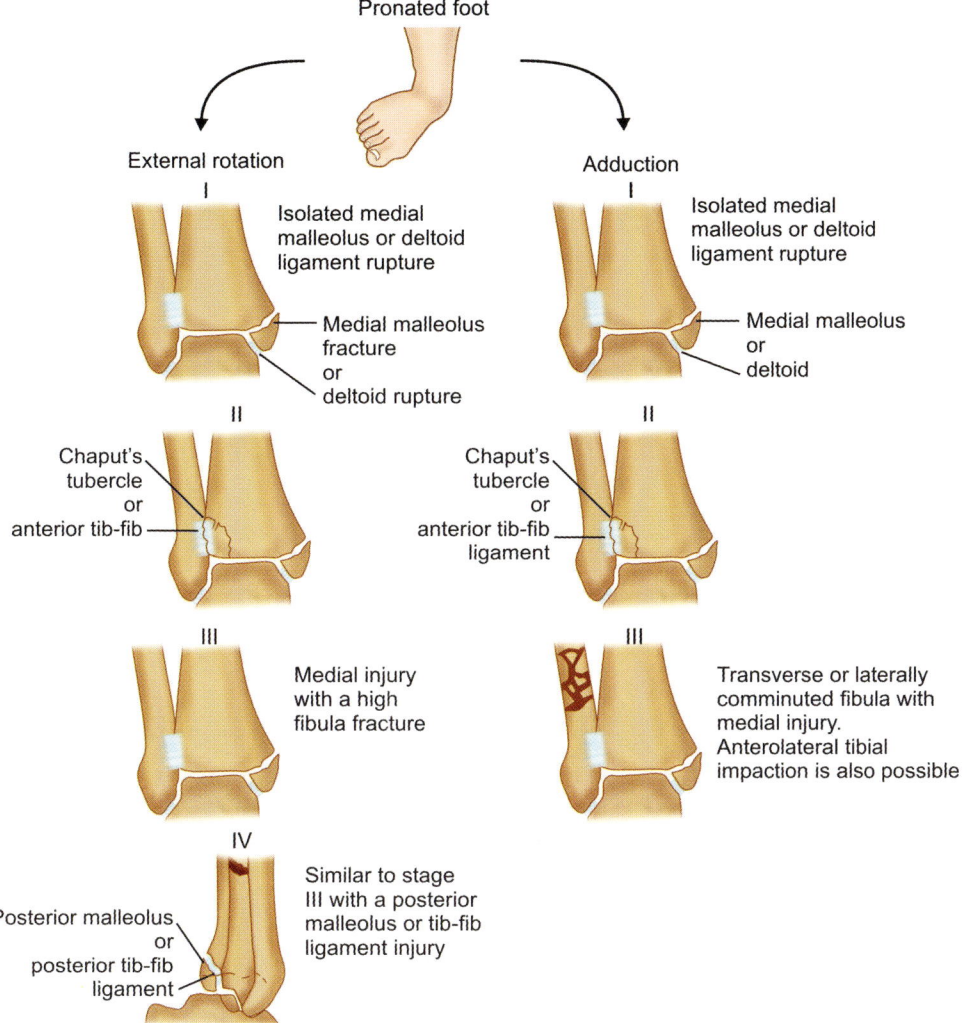

Pronated foot

External rotation

I

Isolated medial
malleolus or deltoid
ligament rupture

Medial malleolus
fracture
or
deltoid rupture

II

Chaput's
tubercle
or
anterior tib-fib

III

Medial injury
with a high
fibula fracture

IV

Posterior malleolus
or
posterior tib-fib
ligament

Similar to stage
III with a posterior
malleolus or tib-fib
ligament injury

Adduction

I

Isolated medial
malleolus or deltoid
ligament rupture

Medial malleolus
or
deltoid

II

Chaput's
tubercle
or
anterior tib-fib
ligament

III

Transverse or laterally
comminuted fibula with
medial injury.
Anterolateral tibial
impaction is also possible

Fig. 4.40: The PER mechanism has four stages of injury and PAB mechanism has three stages.

- *Stage II*: Disruption of the anterior tibio-fibular ligament with or without an avulsion fracture at its insertion sites.
- *Stage III*: Fracture of the fibula occurs through torsion resulting in an oblique or spiral fracture. It differs from SER IV by it is typically suprasyndesmotic (equivalent to Denis-Weber type C) and that the long spike is anterior, PER III is unstable and there is high chances of syndesmotic injury. Maisonneuve fracture variant is seen in this of injury mechanism.
- *Stage IV*: Rupture of the posterior tibio-fibular ligament or an avulsion fracture of the posterolateral tibia.

FOOT

17. TALUS FRACTURE

HAWKINS CLASSIFICATION OF TALAR NECK FRACTURE (Fig. 4.41)

This fractures was first described by Hawkins in 1970. His three-part classification was primarily based on the amount of fracture displacement and provided information on the prognosis for AVN. This classification was later modified by **Canale and Kelly** to include a fourth type.

Type I. Injury is an undisplaced vertical fracture of the talar neck.

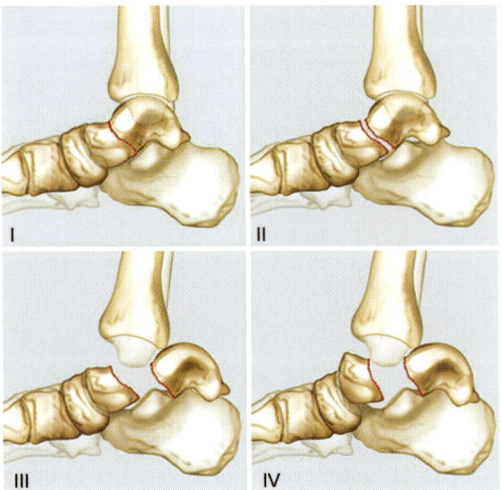

Fig. 4.41: Hawkin's classification of talar neck fractures.

Type II. Fracture is a displaced fracture; the subtalar joint is subluxated or dislocated but the ankle joint is normal.

Type III. Injury is similar to a type II injury, but subluxation or dislocation of both the ankle and subtalar joints occurs.

Type IV. Injury is very rare and is characterized by dislocation of the talar head from the talonavicular joint.

18. CALCANEAL FRACTURE

A. CLASSIFICATION OF EXTRA-ARTICULAR FRACTURES

- *Anterior process fractures*: Due to strong plantar flexion and inversion, which tightens the bifurcate and interosseous ligaments and leads to an avulsion fracture; alternatively, may occur with forefoot abduction with calcaneocuboid compression. Often confused with lateral ankle sprain; seen on lateral or lateral oblique views.
- *Tuberosity fractures*: Due to avulsion by the Achilles tendon, especially in diabetics or osteoporotic women, or, rarely, may result from direct trauma; seen on lateral radiographs.
- *Medial process fractures*: Vertical shear fracture due to loading of the heel in valgus; seen on axial radiograph.

- *Sustentacular fractures*: Occur with heel loading accompanied by severe foot inversion. Often confused with medial ankle sprain; seen on axial radiograph.
- *Body fractures not involving the subtalar articulation*: Due to axial loading. Significant comminution, widening, and loss of height may occur along with a reduction in the Bohler angle without posterior facet involvement.

B. ESSEX LOPRESTI CLASSIFICATION

Details are shown in Fig. 4.42.

C. SOUER AND REMY CLASSIFICATION

Based on the number of bony fragments determined on Broden, lateral, and Harris axial views:

First degree: Nondisplaced shear type intra-articular fractures with widening of joint surface.

Second degree: Secondary fracture lines resulting in a minimum of three additional pieces, with the posterior main fragment breaking into lateral, middle, and medial fragments

Third degree: Highly comminuted that it could not be classified.

D. SANDERS CLASSIFICATION (Fig. 4.43)

- Classification based on the number and location of articular fragments as observed by computed tomography and found on the coronal image that shows the widest surface of the inferior facet of the talus.
- The posterior facet of the calcaneus is divided into three fracture lines (A, B, and C, corresponding to lateral, middle, and medial fracture lines, respectively, on the coronal image).
- Thus, a total of four potential pieces can result: lateral, central, medial, and sustentaculum tali.

Type I. All nondisplaced fractures regardless of the number of fracture lines.

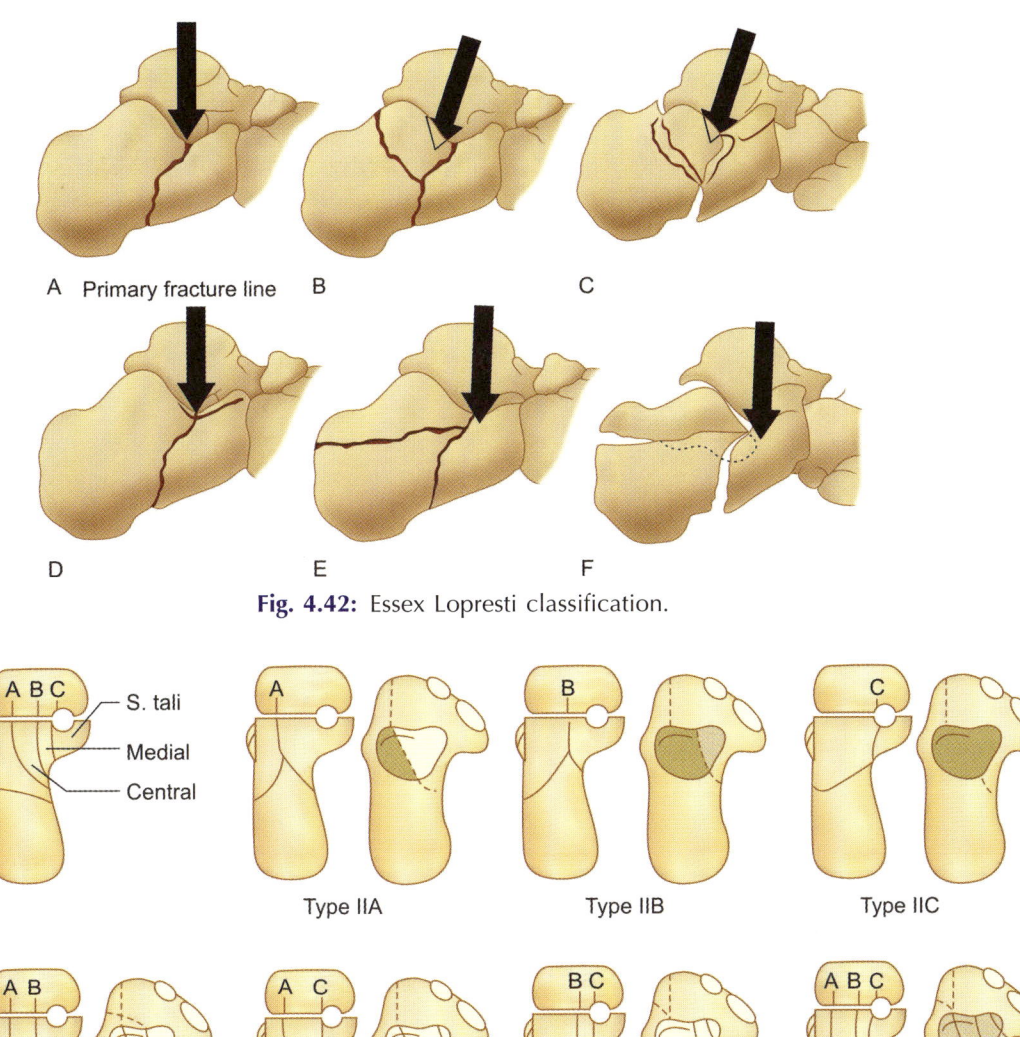

Fig. 4.42: Essex Lopresti classification.

Fig. 4.43: Sanders classification of calcaneal fracture.

Type II. Two-part fractures of the posterior facet; subtypes IIA, IIB, IIC based on the location of the primary fracture line.

Type III. Three-part fractures in which a centrally depressed fragment exists; subtypes IIIAB, IIIAC, IIIBC.

Type IV. Four-part articular fractures; highly comminuted.

FRACTURES OF THE MIDFOOT

19. MIDTARSAL JOINT (CHOPART JOINT) MAIN AND JOWETT CLASSIFICATION

1. *Medial stress injury*
- This is an inversion injury with adduction of the midfoot on the hindfoot.
- Flake fractures of the dorsal margin of the talus or navicular and of the lateral margin

of the calcaneus or the cuboid may indicate a sprain.

- In more severe injuries, the midfoot may be completely dislocated or an isolated talonavicular dislocation may occur. A medial swivel dislocation is one in which the talonavicular joint is dislocated, the subtalar joint is subluxed, and the calcaneocuboid joint is intact.

2. *Longitudinal stress injury*

- Force is transmitted through the metatarsal heads proximally along the rays, with resultant compression of the midfoot between the metatarsals and the talus with the foot plantar flexed.
- Longitudinal forces pass between the cuneiforms and fracture the navicular, typically in a vertical pattern.

3. *Lateral stress injury*

- This stress injury called "nutcracker fracture" is a characteristic fracture of the cuboid as the forefoot is driven laterally, causing crushing of the cuboid between the calcaneus and the bases of the fourth and fifth metatarsals.
- This is most commonly an avulsion fracture of the navicular with a comminuted compression fracture of the cuboid.
- In more severe trauma, the talonavicular joint subluxes laterally and the lateral column of the foot collapses due to comminution of the calcaneocuboid joint.

4. *Plantar stress injury*: Plantarly directed forces may result in sprains to the midtarsal region with avulsion fractures of the dorsal lip of the navicular, talus, or anterior process of the calcaneus.

5. *Crush injuries.*

20. NAVICULAR FRACTURES

A. EICHENHOLTZ AND LEVINE CLASSIFICATION

Type I. Avulsion fractures of tuberosity

Type II. A fracture involving the dorsal lip

Type III. A fracture through the body.

B. SANGEORZAN CLASSIFICATION (Fig. 4.44)

Type I. Transverse fracture line in the coronal plane, with no angulation of the forefoot.

Type II. The major fracture line from dorsolateral to plantar medial with talonavicular joint disruption and forefoot is displaced laterally.

Type III. Comminuted fracture pattern with naviculo-cuneiform joint disruption; associated fractures may exist (cuboid, anterior calcaneus, calcaneocuboid joints).

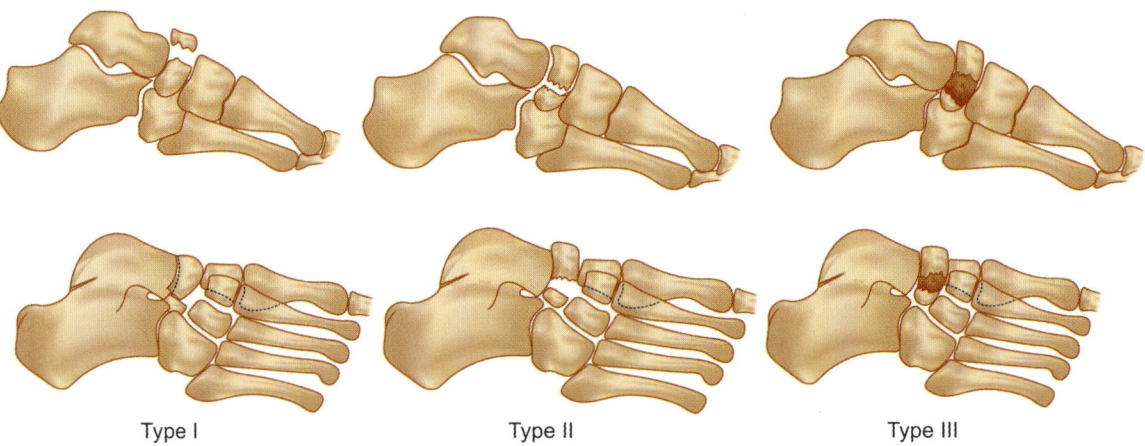

Type I   Type II   Type III

Fig. 4.44: Sangeorzan classification.

21. CUBOID FRACTURES

OTA CLASSIFICATION OF CUBOID FRACTURES

Higher letters and numbers denote more significant injury.

Type A. Extra-articular
- *Type A1.* Extra-articular, avulsion
- *Type A2.* Extra-articular, coronal
- *Type A3.* Extra-articular, multifragmentary

Type B. Partial articular, single joint (calcaneocuboid or cubotarsal)
- *Type B1.* Partial articular, sagittal
- *Type B2.* Partial articular, horizontal

Type C. Articular, calcaneocuboid and cubotarsal involvement
- *Type C1.* Articular, multifragmentary
- *Type C1.1.* Nondisplaced
- *Type C1.2.* Displaced.

22. TARSOMETATARSAL (LISFRANC) JOINT

Stages of injury (Fig. 4.45): Nunley and Vertullo reported staging system based on weight bearing radiographic analysis.

A. QUENU AND KUSS CLASSIFICATION (Fig. 4.46)

Based on commonly observed patterns of injury.

Type 1. Homolateral. All five metatarsals displaced in the same direction.

Type 2. Isolated. One or two metatarsals displaced form the others.

Type 3. Divergent. Displacement of the metatarsals in both the sagittal and coronal planes.

B. MYERSON CLASSIFICATION (Fig. 4.47)

A. Total incongruity
    A1. Lateral
    A2. Dorsoplantar

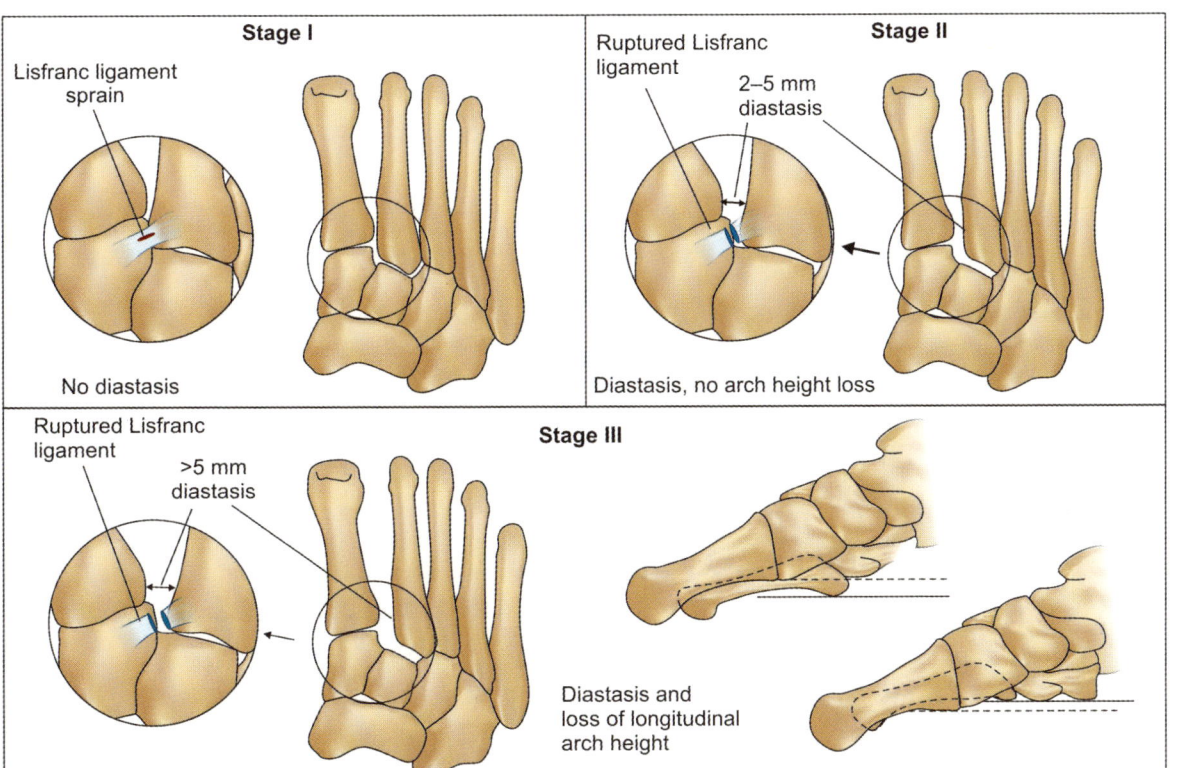

Fig. 4.45: Nunley and Vertullo staging system of lisfranc fracture dislocation.

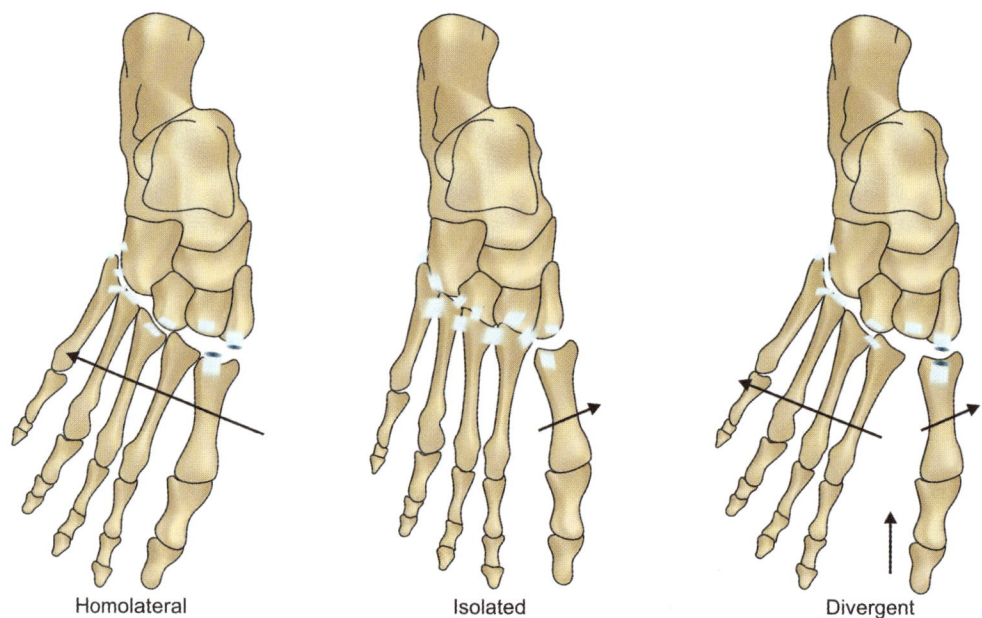

Fig. 4.46: Quenu and Kuss classification of Lisfranc fracture dislocation.

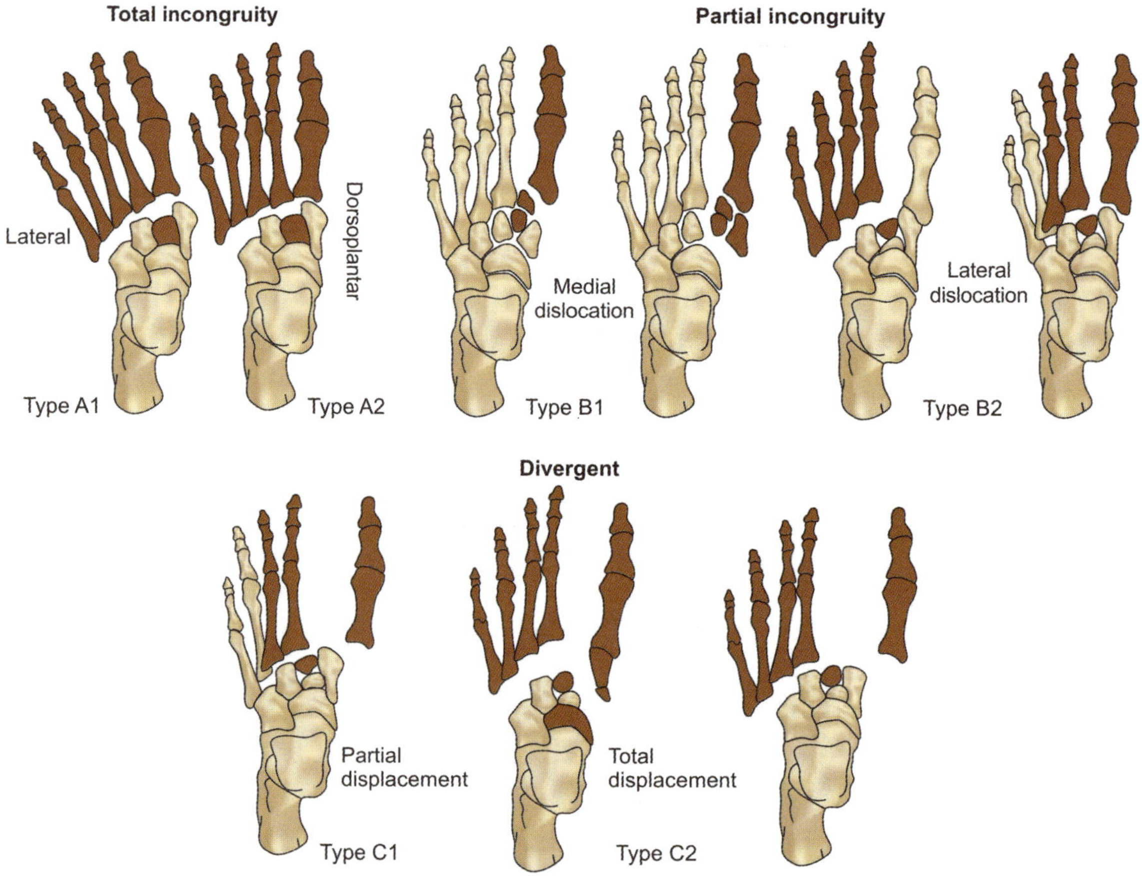

Fig. 4.47: Myerson classification.

B. Partial incongruity
  B1. Medial dislocation
  B2. Lateral dislocation

C. Divergent
  C1. Partial displacement
  C2. Total displacement

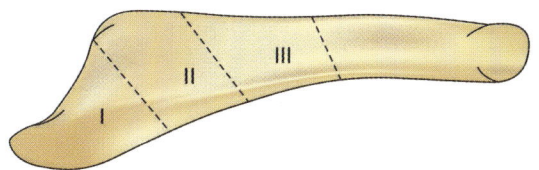

Fig. 4.49: Zonal division of the base of fifth metatarsal

23. FRACTURES OF THE BASE OF THE FIFTH METATARSAL

DAMERON CLASSIFICATION (Figs 4.48 and 4.49)

Zone I. Avulsion fractures (pseudo-Jones fracture)

Zone II. Fractures at the metaphyseal-diaphyseal junction (Jones fracture)

Zone III. Stress fractures of the proximal 1.5 cm of the shaft of the fifth metatarsal.

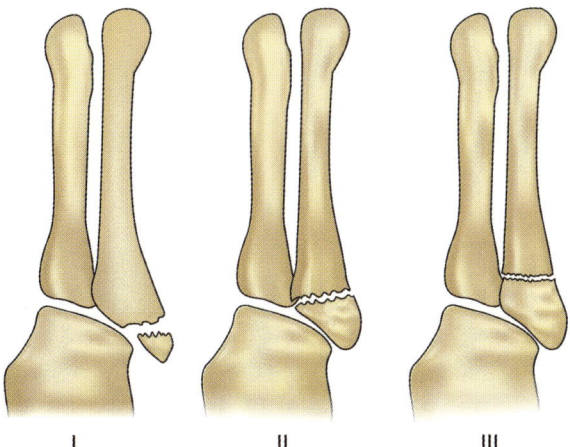

Fig. 4.48: Dameron and Lawrence and Boote classification.

24. FIRST METATARSOPHALANGEAL JOINT

BOWERS AND MARTIN CLASSIFICATION

Grade I. Strain at the proximal attachment of the volar plate from the first metatarsal head.

Grade II. Avulsion of the volar plate from the metatarsal head.

Grade III. Impaction injury to the dorsal surface of the metatarsal head with or without an avulsion or chip fracture.

25. DISLOCATION OF THE FIRST METATARSOPHALANGEAL JOINT

JAHSS CLASSIFICATION

Based on integrity of the sesamoid complex:

Type I. Volar plate is avulsed off the first metatarsal head; proximal phalanx displaced dorsally; intersesamoid ligament remains intact and lies over the dorsum of the meta-tarsal head.

Type II
- *Type IIA.* Intersesamoid ligament is ruptured
- *Type IIB.* Longitudinal fracture of either sesamoid is seen.

Spine

CERVICAL SPINE

1. INJURIES TO THE OCCIPUT C1–C2 COMPLEX

A. Anderson and Montesano Classification of Occipital Condyle Fractures (Fig. 5.1)

The fractures can be subdivided into three types based on the morphology and mechanism of injury:

Type I fracture (~15%)
- Impaction fracture of the occipital condyle
- Due to axial compression
- Stable injury

Type II fracture (~50%)
- Basilar skull fracture that extends to involve the occipital condyle
- Due to a direct blow to the skull
- Stable injury

Type III fracture (~35%)
- Avulsion injury of the condyle in the region of alar ligament attachment
- Due to forced contralateral bending and rotation
- Potentially unstable injury

Type I and type II injuries are generally stable because the alar ligament and tectorial membrane are preserved, while type 3 is potentially unstable.

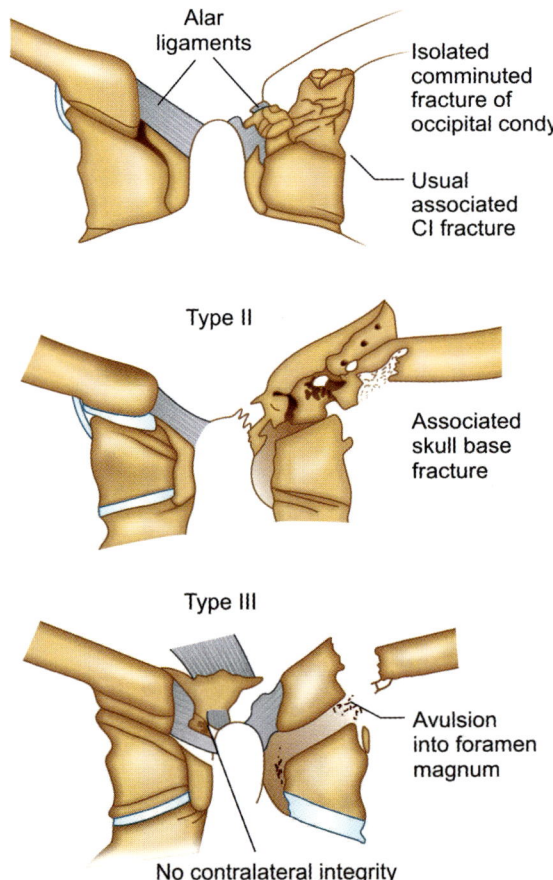

Type I

Alar ligaments

Isolated comminuted fracture of occipital condyle

Usual associated CI fracture

Type II

Associated skull base fracture

Type III

Avulsion into foramen magnum

No contralateral integrity

Fig. 5.1: Illustration of the types of occipital condyle fracture according to the classification of Anderson and Montesano, which is the most widely used and divides these fractures into three types.

B. Atlanto-occipital Dislocation (Craniovertebral Dissociation)

TABLE 5.1: Traynelis classification (direction of displacement) (Fig. 5.2)

Type I	Anterior occiput dislocation
Type II	Longitudinal dislocation
Type III	Posterior occiput dislocation

TABLE 5.2: Harbourview classification system (degree of instability)

Stage I	Minimal or non-displaced, unilateral injury to craniocervical ligaments	Stable
Stage II	Minimally displaced, but MRI demonstrates significant soft-tissue injuries. Stability may be based on traction test	Stable or Unstable
Stage III	Gross craniocervical misalignment (BAI or BDI >2 mm beyond normal limits)	Unstable

C. Atlas Fractures

Levine and Edwards Classification

1. Burst fracture (Jefferson fracture). Axial load injury resulting in four fractures: two in the posterior arch and two in the anterior arch.
2. Posterior arch fractures. Hyperextension injury that is associated with odontoid and axis fractures.
3. Comminuted fractures. Axial load and lateral bending injury associated with high nonunion rate and poor clinical result.
4. Anterior arch fractures. Hyperextension injury.
5. Lateral mass fractures. Axial load and lateral bending injury.
6. Transverse process fracture. Avulsion injury.
7. Inferior tubercle fracture. Avulsion of the longus colli muscle.

D. Atlantoaxial Rotatory Subluxation and Dislocation

Fielding Classification (Fig. 5.3)

Type I. Simple rotatory displacement without anterior shift. Odontoid acts as a pivot point; transverse ligament intact.

Type II. Rotatory displacement with anterior displacement of 3.5 mm. Opposite facet acts as a pivot; transverse ligament insufficient.

Type III. Rotatory displacement with anterior displacement of more than 5 mm. Both joints anteriorly subluxed. Transverse and alar ligaments incompetent.

Type IV. Rare; both joints posteriorly subluxed.

Type V. (Levine and Edwards) frank dislocation; extremely rare.

E. Fractures of the Odontoid Process (DENS)

Anderson and D'Alonzo Classification (Table 5.3 and Fig. 5.4)

TABLE 5.3: Anderson and D'Alonzo classification

Type I (5%)	Oblique avulsion fx of tip of odontoid. Due to avulsion of alar ligament. Although rare, atlanto-occipital instability should be ruled out with flexion and extension films	Stable
Type II (60%)	Fx through waist (high non-union rate due to interruption of blood supply)	Unstable
Type III (30%)	Fx extends into cancellous body of C2 and involves a variable portion of the C1–C2 joint	Stable

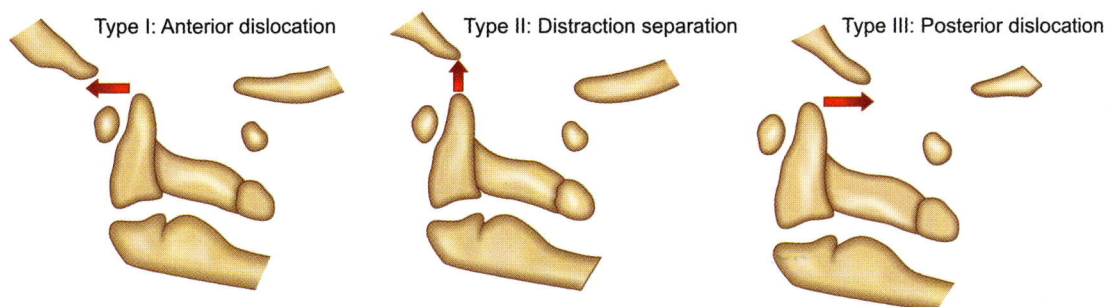

Fig. 5.2: Traynelis classification (direction of displacement).

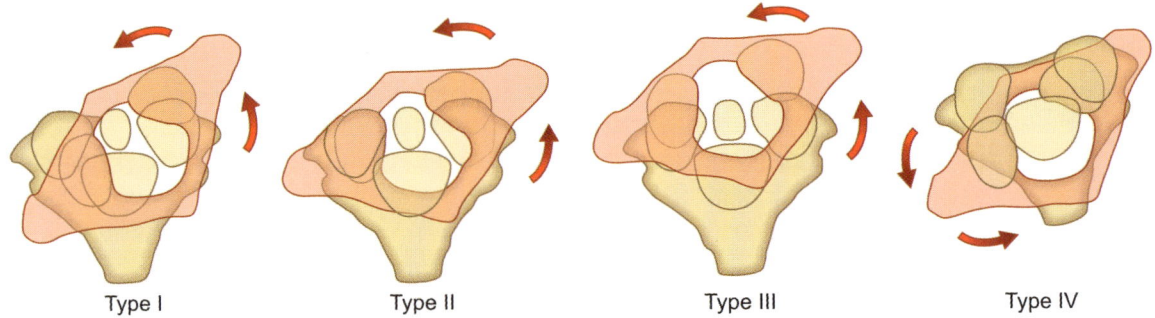

Type I   Type II   Type III   Type IV

Fig. 5.3: Fielding classification for atlantoaxial rotatory subluxation and dislocation.

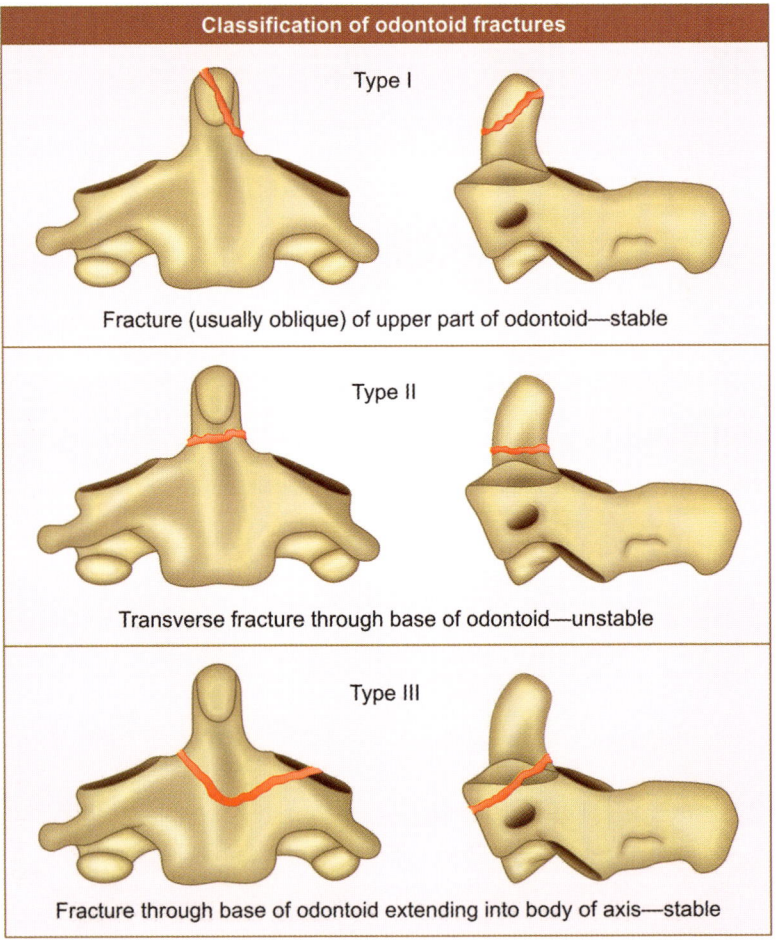

Classification of odontoid fractures

Type I

Fracture (usually oblique) of upper part of odontoid—stable

Type II

Transverse fracture through base of odontoid—unstable

Type III

Fracture through base of odontoid extending into body of axis—stable

Fig. 5.4: Anderson and D'Alonzo classification of odontoid fractures.

F. Traumatic Spondylolisthesis of Axis (Hangman's Fracture)

Levine and Edwards (Fig. 5.5)

Type I. Minimally displaced with no angulation; translation <3 mm; stable.

Type II. Significant angulation at C2–C3; translation >3 mm; unstable; C2–C3 disc disrupted. Subclassified into flexion, extension, and listhetic types.

Type IIA: Avulsion of entire C2–C3 intervertebral disc in flexion, leaving the anterior

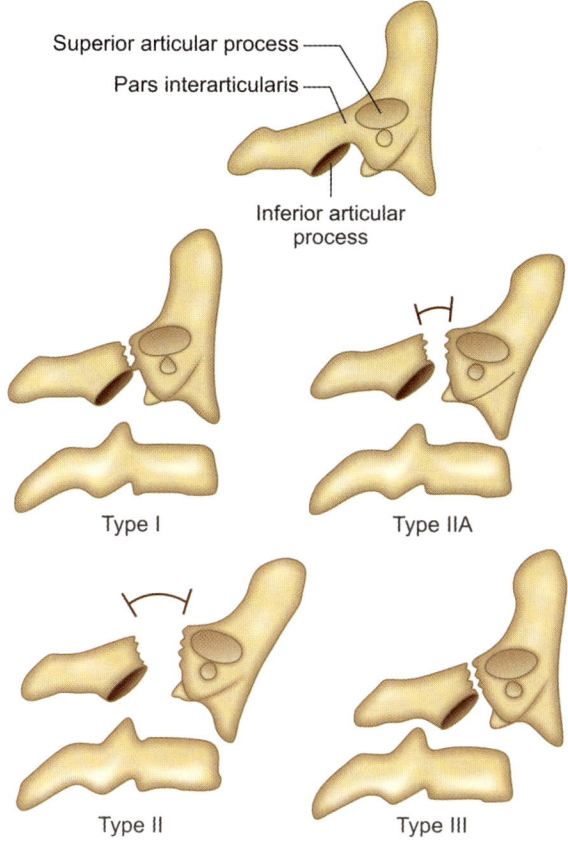

Superior articular process
Pars interarticularis
Inferior articular process

Type I   Type IIA

Type II   Type III

Fig. 5.5: Levine and Edward classification for Hangman's fracture.

longitudinal ligament intact. Results in severe angulation. No translation; unstable due to flexion-distraction injury.

Type III. Rare; results from initial anterior facet dislocation of C2 on C3 followed by extension injury fracturing the neural arch. Results in severe angulation and translation with unilateral or bilateral facet dislocation of C2–C3; unstable.

2. INJURIES TO C3–C7

Allen Classification (Fig. 5.6)

1. Compressive Flexion (Shear Mechanism Resulting in "Teardrop" Fractures)

Stage I. Blunting of anterior body; posterior element intact.

Stage II. "Beaking" of the anterior body; loss of anterior vertebral height.

TABLE 5.4: Allen and Ferguson classification of subaxial spine injuries

1. Flexion-compression	
2. Vertical compression	
3. Flexion-distraction	Stage 1: Facet subluxation
	Stage 2: Unilateral facet dislocation
	Stage 3: Bilateral facet dislocation with 50% displacement
	Stage 4: Complete dislocation (100% displacement)
4. Extension-compression	
5. Extension-distraction	
6. Lateral flexion	

Stage III. Fracture line passing from anterior body through the inferior subchondral plate.

Stage IV. Inferoposterior margin displaced <3 mm into the spinal canal.

Stage V. Teardrop fracture; inferoposterior margin >3 mm into the spinal canal; posterior ligaments and the posterior longitudinal ligament have failed.

2. Vertical Compression (Burst Fractures)

Stage I. Fracture through superior or inferior endplate with no displacement.

Stage II. Fracture through both endplates with minimal displacement.

Stage III. Burst fracture; displacement of fragments peripherally and into the neural canal.

3. Distractive Flexion (Dislocations)

Stage I. Failure of the posterior ligaments, divergence of spinous processes, and facet subluxation.

Stage II. Unilateral facet dislocation; displacement is always <50%.

Stage III. Bilateral facet dislocation; displacement >50%.

Stage IV. Bilateral facet dislocation with 100% translation.

4. Compressive Extension

Stage I. Unilateral vertebral arch fracture.

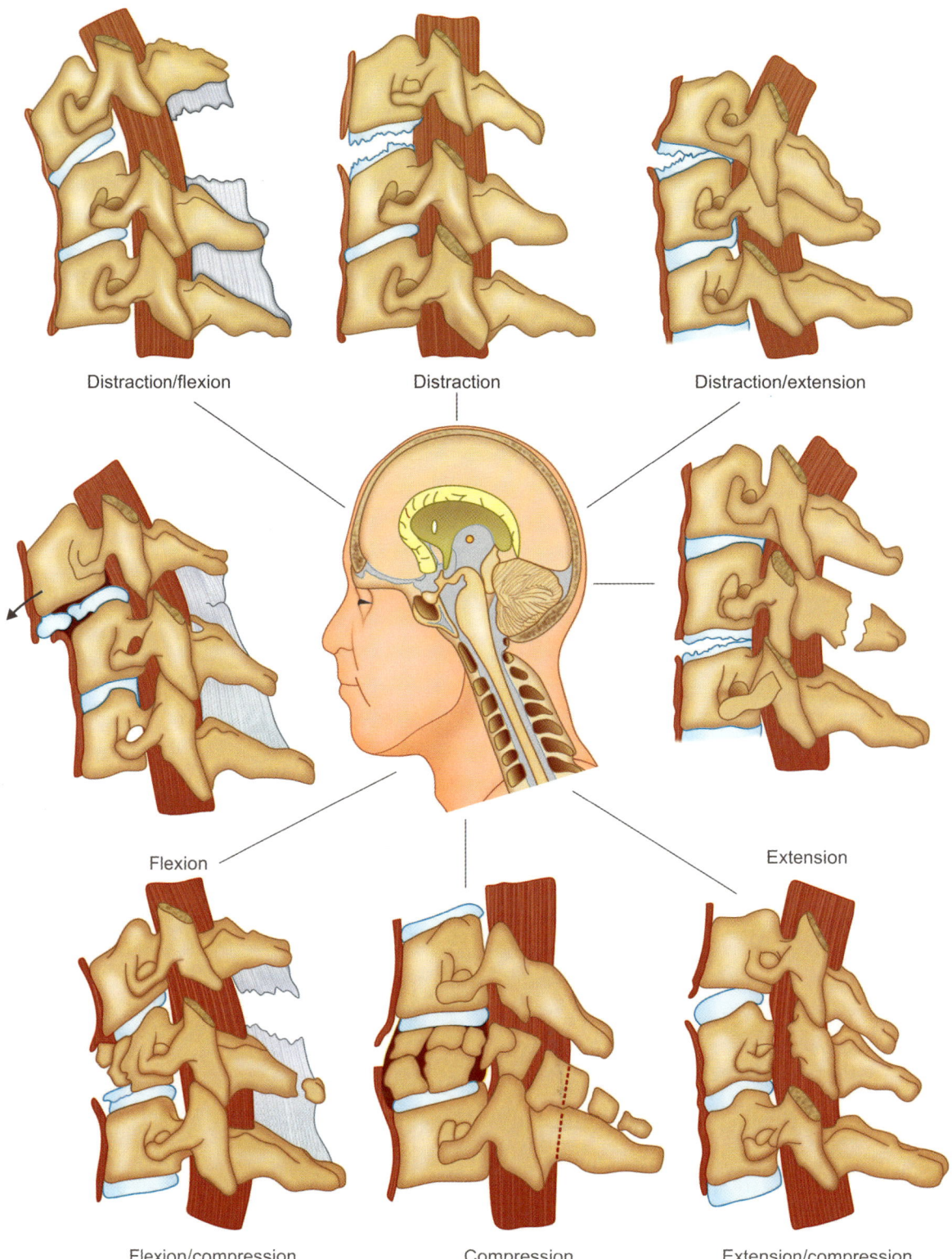

Distraction/flexion   Distraction   Distraction/extension

Flexion   Extension

Flexion/compression   Compression   Extension/compression

Fig. 5.6: Allen classification for fractures C3–C7.

Stage II. Bilaminar fracture without other tissue failure.

Stage III. Bilateral vertebral arch fracture with fracture of the articular processes, pedicles, and lamina without vertebral body displacement.

Stage IV. Bilateral vertebral arch fracture with full vertebral body displacement anteriorly; ligamentous failure at the posterosuperior and anteroinferior margins.

5. Distractive Extension

Stage I. Failure of anterior ligamentous complex or transverse fracture of the body; widening of the disc space and no posterior displacement.

Stage II. Failure of posterior ligament complex with displacement of the vertebral body into the canal.

6. Lateral Flexion

Stage I. Asymmetric unilateral compression fracture of the vertebral body plus a vertebral arch fracture on the ipsilateral side without displacement.

Stage II. Displacement of the arch on the anteroposterior view or failure of the ligaments on the contralateral side with articular process separation.

3. ORTHOPEDIC TRAUMA ASSOCIATION (OTA)

Classification of Cervical Spine Injuries (Fig. 5.7)

Type A. Compression injuries of the body (compressive forces)
- *Type A1.* Impaction fractures
- *Type A2.* Split fractures
- *Type A3.* Burst fractures

Type B. Distraction injuries of the anterior and posterior elements (tensile forces)
- *Type B1.* Posterior disruption predominantly osseous, i.e. disruption occurs through fractured bony structures only (flexion–distraction injury).

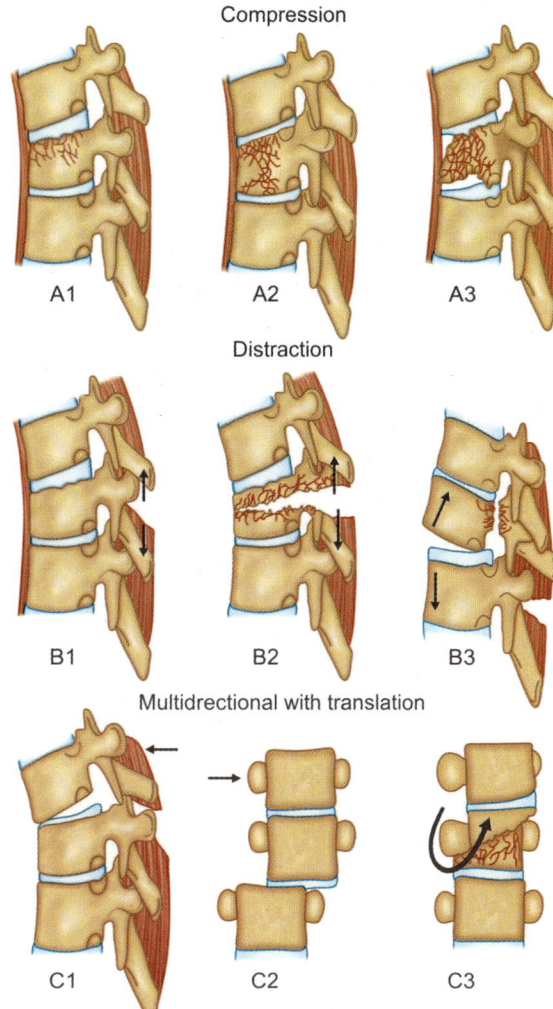

Fig. 5.7: OTA classification for cervical spine injuries

- *Type B2.* Posterior distraction injury with complete disruption of posterior capsuloligamentous complex together with vertebral body, disc and/or facet injury (flexion–distraction injury).
- *Type B3.* Anterior disruption through the disk (hyperextension-shear injury)

Type C. Multidirectional injuries with translation affecting the anterior and posterior elements (axial torque causing rotation injuries)
- *Type C1.* Rotational wedge, split, and burst fractures
- *Type C2.* Flexion subluxation with rotation
- *Type C3.* Rotational shear injuries (Holdsworth slice rotation fracture).

4. THORACOLUMBAR SPINE FRACTURES

A. McAfee Classification (Fig. 5.8)

Classification is based on the failure mode of the middle osteoligamentous complex (posterior longitudinal ligament, posterior half of the vertebral body, and posterior annulus fibrosus:

The six injury patterns are the following:
1. Wedge-compression fracture
2. Stable burst fracture
3. Unstable burst fracture
4. Chance fracture
5. Flexion-distraction injury
6. Translational injuries.

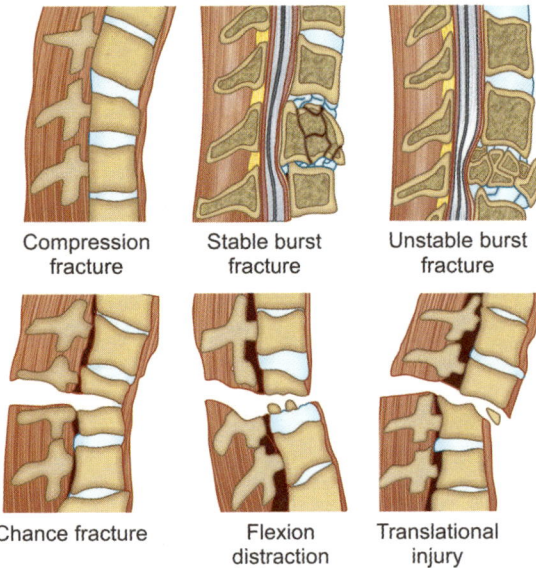

Compression fracture   Stable burst fracture   Unstable burst fracture

Chance fracture   Flexion distraction   Translational injury

Fig. 5.8: McAfee classification for thoracolumbar spine injuries.

B. Denis Classification

The three-column model according to Denis (Fig. 5.9):

Anterior column
• Anterior longitudinal ligament
• Anterior half of vertebral body
• Anterior portion of annulus fibrosis

Middle column
• Posterior longitudinal ligament
• Posterior half of vertebral body
• Posterior aspect of annulus fibrosis

Posterior column
• Neural arch
• Ligamentum flavum
• Facet capsule
• Interspinous ligament
   Based on the three-column model, fractures are classified according to the mechanism of injury and the resulting fracture pattern into one of the following categories:
1. Compression
2. Burst
3. Flexion distraction
4. Fracture dislocation

1. Compression Fractures (Fig. 5.10)

Four subtypes described on the basis of endplate involvement are as follows:
Type A. Fracture of both endplates
Type B. Fractures of the superior endplate
Type C. Fractures of the inferior endplate
Type D. Both endplates intact

2. Burst Fractures (Fig. 5.11)

Failure under axial load of both the anterior and middle column originating at the level

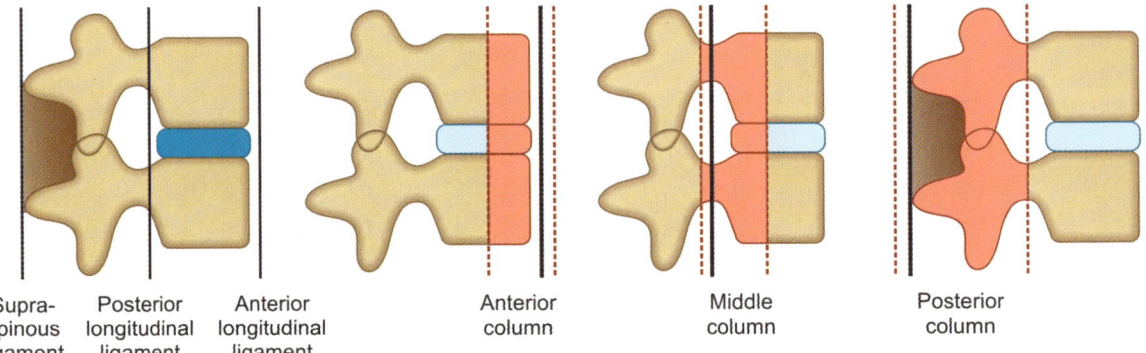

Supra-spinous ligament   Posterior longitudinal ligament   Anterior longitudinal ligament   Anterior column   Middle column   Posterior column

Fig. 5.9: Denis' concept of three-column model.

Compression Fractures

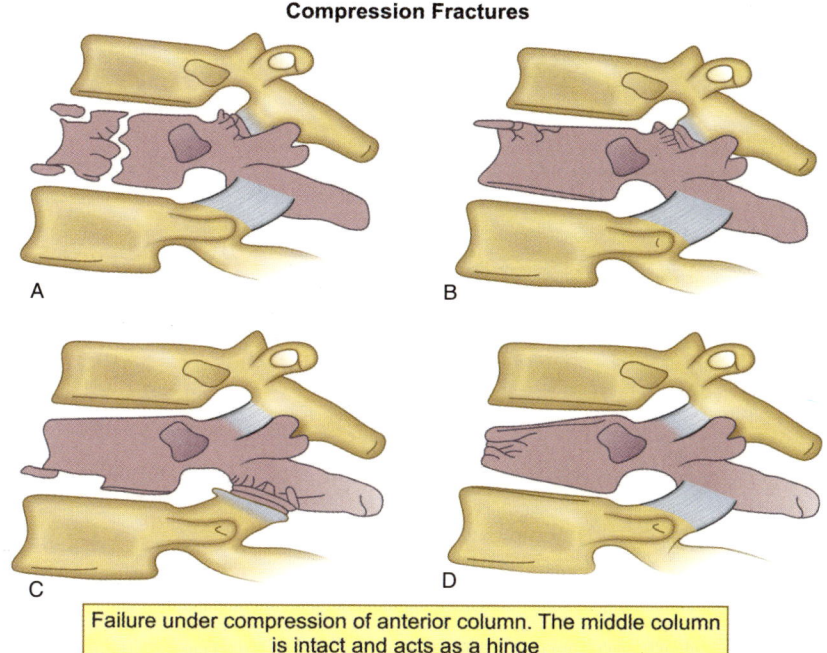

Failure under compression of anterior column. The middle column is intact and acts as a hinge

Fig. 5.10: Pictorial representation of compression fracture.

Burst Fractures

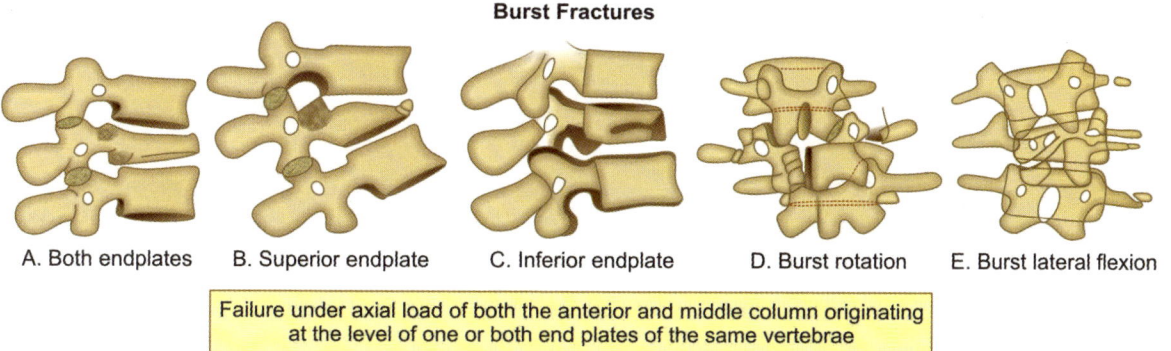

| A. Both endplates | B. Superior endplate | C. Inferior endplate | D. Burst rotation | E. Burst lateral flexion |

Failure under axial load of both the anterior and middle column originating at the level of one or both end plates of the same vertebrae

Fig. 5.11: Burst thoracolumbar spine fractures.

of one or both the end plates of the same vertebrae.

Type A. Fractures of both endplates

Type B. Fracture of the superior endplate

Type C. Fracture of the inferior endplate

Type D. Burst rotation

Type E. Burst lateral flexion

Criteria for unstable burst fracture

- Neurologic deficit
- Posterior element injuries

- Loss of more than 50% of anterior vertebral body height
- Greater than 25 to 35 deg of kyphosis
- Thoracolumbar burst fracture:
  - Angulation of thoracolumbar junction >20°
  - Canal comprimise >30 percent.

3. Flexion–distraction Injuries (Chance Fractures, Seat Belt Type Injuries) (Fig. 5.12)

Type A. One-level bony injury (Fig. 5.13)

Type B. One-level ligamentous

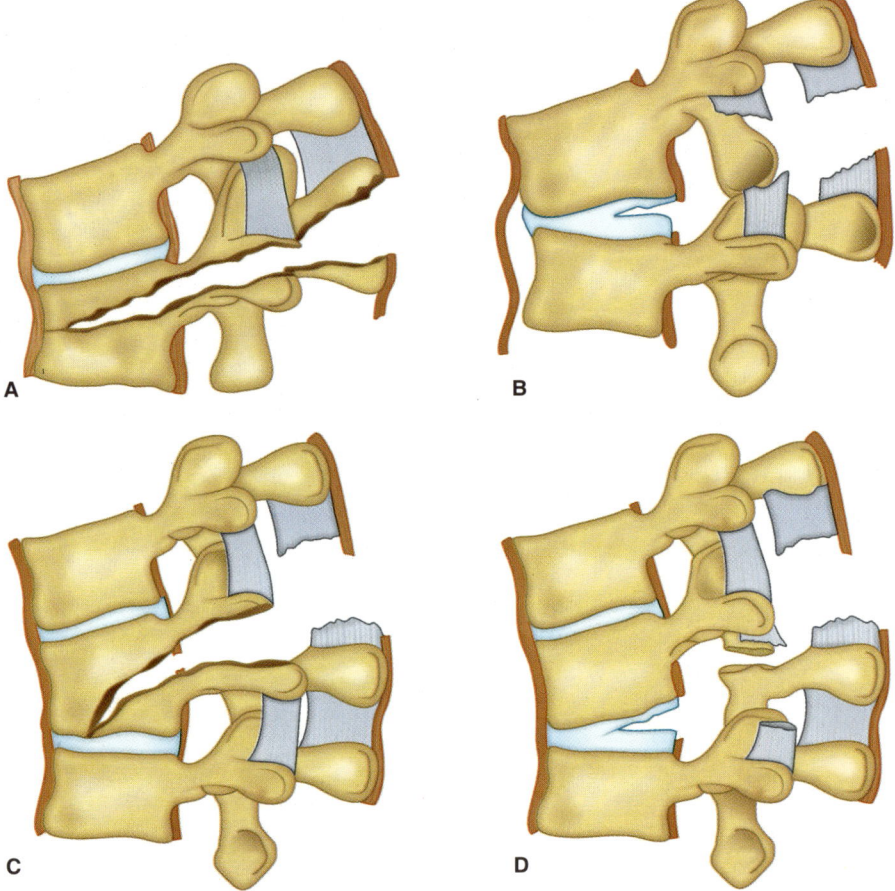

Fig. 5.12: Pictorial representation of flexion distraction injury.

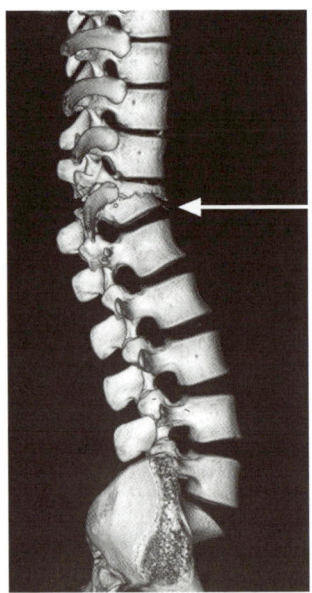

Fig. 5.13: 3D-CT showing chance fracture.

Type C. Two-level injury through bony middle column

Type D. Two-level injury through ligamentous middle column.

4. Fracture Dislocations (Fig. 5.14)

Type A. Flexion–rotation. Posterior and middle column fail in tension and rotation; anterior column fails in compression and rotation; 75% have neurological deficits, 52% of these are complete lesions.

Type B. Shear failure of all three columns, most commonly in the posteroanterior direction; all cases with complete neurological deficits.

Type C. Flexion–distraction. Tension failure of posterior and middle columns, with anterior tear of annulus fibrosus and stripping of the

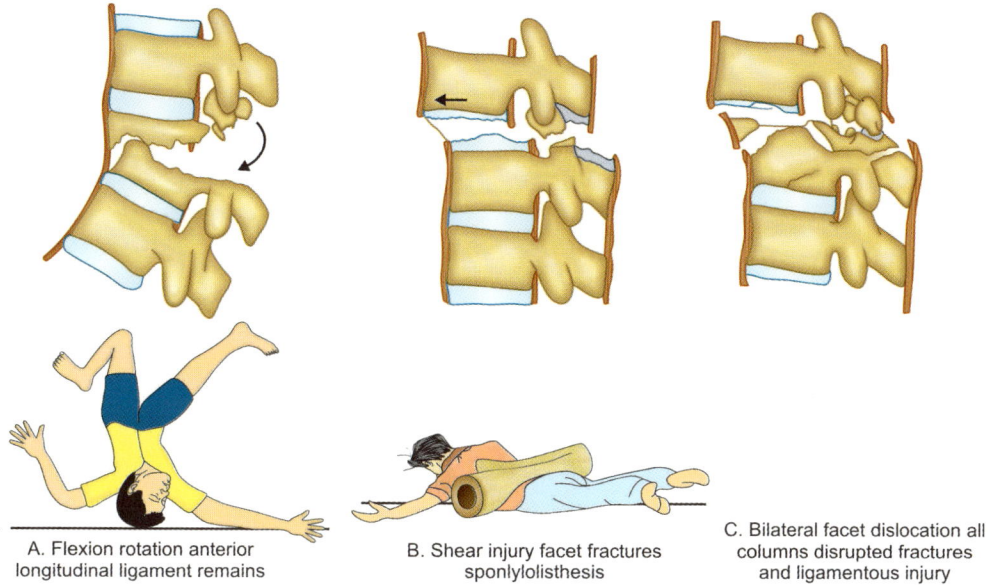

A. Flexion rotation anterior
longitudinal ligament remains

B. Shear injury facet fractures
sponlylolisthesis

C. Bilateral facet dislocation all
columns disrupted fractures
and ligamentous injury

Fig. 5.14: Pictorial representation of fracture dislocation.

anterior longitudinal ligament; 75% with neurological deficits (all incomplete).

C. Thoracolumbar Injury Classification and Severity (TLICS) Scale (Table 5.5)

The score was given by Vaccaro et al and the total score is determined by adding the assigned points in all the major categories. Determination of the total points is designed to help surgeons and nonsurgeons assess the severity of the injury and to guide the decision-between operative and nonoperative manage-ment. Patients with ≤3 total points are considered nonoperative candidates, whereas patients with ≥5 points are operative candidates. Patients with a total score of 4 fall into an indistinct category, where either nonoperative or operative treatment may be considered.

D. White and Panjabi Criteria: Spine Instability

- Anterior elements destroyed or unable to function = 2
- Posterior elements destroyed or unable to function = 2
- Positive stretch test = 2 (7.5 degree angulation with 25 pound extraction)

Dynamic flexion–extension radiographs
- Sagittal translation >3.5 mm or 20% of vertebra = 2
- Sagittal rotation >11 degree = 2

On resting static radiographs
- Sagittal plane displacement 3.5 mm or 20%
- Relative sagittal plane angulation >20 degrees.
- Developmentally narrow spinal canal sagittal diameter <13 mm or Torg–Pavlov ratio <0.8.
- Spinal cord damage = 2
- Nerve root damage = 1
- Abnormal disc narrowing = 1
- Dangerous loads anticipated = 1
  - The fracture is unstable if the total score is ≥5.

TABLE 5.5: TLIC scale

Morphology	Qualifier	Points
Compression		1
Burst		+1
Translational/rotational		3
Distraction		4
Neurologic status	**Qualifier**	**Points**
Intact		0
Nerve root		2
Cord conus medullaris	Incomplete	3
	Complete	2
Cauda equina		3
Posterior ligamentous complex		**Points**
Intact		0
Injury suspected/indeterminate		2
Injured		3

E. ASIA Impairment Scale (Fig. 5.15)

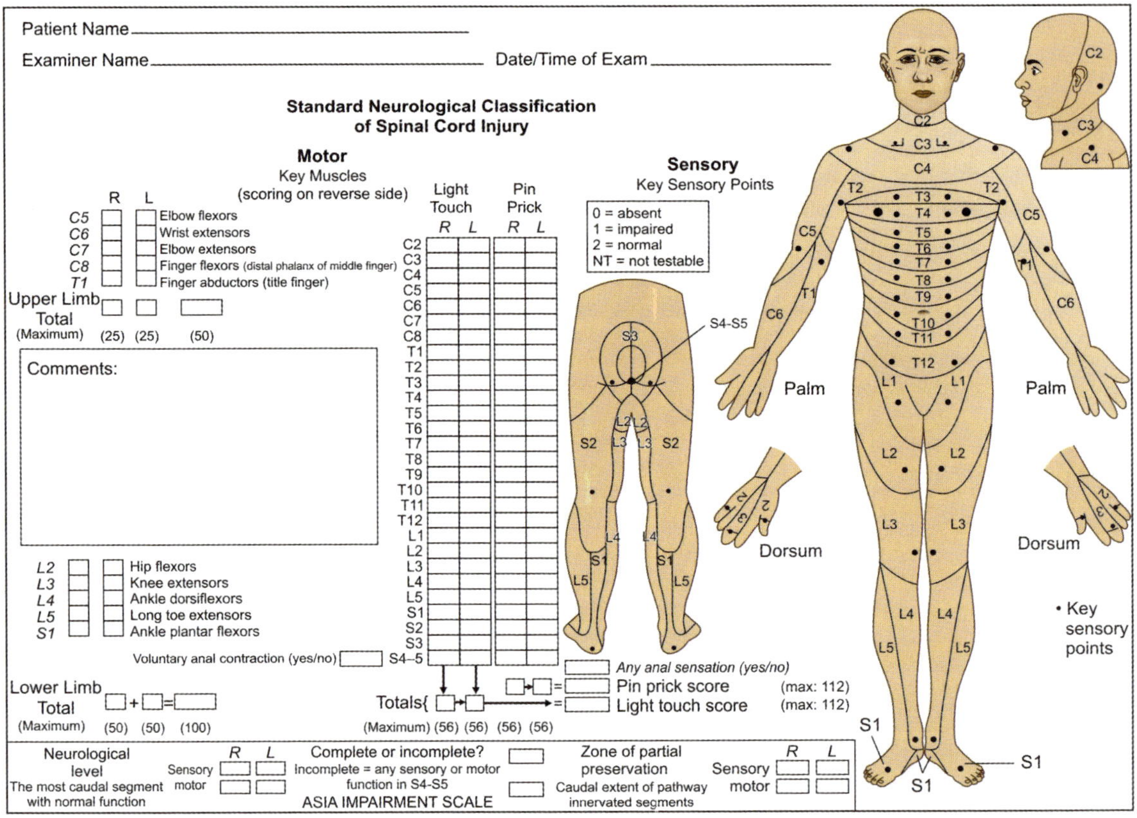

Patient Name _____

Examiner Name _____ Date/Time of Exam _____

Standard Neurological Classification of Spinal Cord Injury

Motor
Key Muscles (scoring on reverse side)

	R	L	
C5	☐	☐	Elbow flexors
C6	☐	☐	Wrist extensors
C7	☐	☐	Elbow extensors
C8	☐	☐	Finger flexors (distal phalanx of middle finger)
T1	☐	☐	Finger abductors (title finger)

Upper Limb ☐ ☐ ☐
Total
(Maximum) (25) (25) (50)

Comments:

	R	L	
L2	☐	☐	Hip flexors
L3	☐	☐	Knee extensors
L4	☐	☐	Ankle dorsiflexors
L5	☐	☐	Long toe extensors
S1	☐	☐	Ankle plantar flexors

Voluntary anal contraction (yes/no) ☐

Lower Limb ☐ + ☐ = ☐
Total
(Maximum) (50) (50) (100)

Sensory
Key Sensory Points

Light Touch   Pin Prick
R L   R L

0 = absent
1 = impaired
2 = normal
NT = not testable

(Segments C2 through S4–5 listed down center column)

Any anal sensation (yes/no) ☐
Pin prick score   (max: 112)
Light touch score   (max: 112)

Totals{ ☐ + ☐ = ☐ }
(Maximum) (56) (56) (56) (56)

Neurological level		R	L
The most caudal segment with normal function	Sensory	☐	☐
	motor	☐	☐

Complete or incomplete? ☐
Incomplete = any sensory or motor function in S4-S5
ASIA IMPAIRMENT SCALE

Zone of partial preservation		R	L
Caudal extent of pathway innervated segments	Sensory	☐	☐
	motor	☐	☐

Palm   Dorsum   • Key sensory points

Muscle Grading

0 total paralysis
1 palpable or visible contraction
2 active movement, full range of motion, gravity eliminated
3 active movement, full range of motion, against gravity
4 active movement, full range of motion, against gravity and provides some resistance
5 active movement, full range of motion, against gravity and provides normal resistance
5* muscle able to exert, in examiner's judgement, sufficient resistance to be considered normal if identifiable inhibiting factors were not present
NT not testable. Patient unable to reliably exert effort or muscle unavailable for testing due to factors such as immobilization, pain on effort or contracture

Asia Impairment Scale

☐ A = **Complete:** No motor or sensory function is preserved in the sacral segment S4–S5.

☐ B = **Incomplete:** Sensory but not motor function is preserved below the neurological level and includes the sacral segment S4–S5.

☐ C = **Incomplete:** Motor function is preserved below the neurological level, and more than half of key muscles below the neurological level have a muscle below the neurological level have a muscle grade less than 3.

☐ D = **Incomplete:** Motor function is preserved below the neurological level, and at least half of key muscles below the neurological level have a muscle grade of 3 or more.

☐ E = **Normal:** Motor and sensory function are normal.

Clinical Syndromes (Optional)

☐ Central cord
☐ Brown-Sequard
☐ Anterior cord
☐ Conus medullaris
☐ Cauda equina

Steps in Classification

The following under is recommended in determining the classification of individuals with SCI.

1. Determine sensory levels for right and left sides.
2. Determine motor levels for right and left sides.
   Note: In regions where there is no myotonic to test, the motor level is preserved to be the same as the sensory level.
3. Determine the single neurological level.
   This is the lowest segment where motor and sensory function is normal on both sides, and is the most cephalad of the sensory and motor levels determined in steps 1 and 2.
4. Determine whether the injury is Complete or Incomplete (sacral sparing).
   If voluntary and contraction = No AND all 54-5 sensory scores = 0 AND any anal sensation = No, then injury to complete. Otherwise injury is incomplete.
5. Determine ASIA Impairment Scale (AIS) Grade

Is injury complete?   If **YES**, ASI=A Record ZPP
NO ↓   (For ZPP record lowest dermatome or
                            myotonic on each side with soem
                            (non-zero score) preservation)

Is injury motor Incomplete?   If **NO**, AIS=B
YES ↓   (Yes=voluntary and contraction OK
                            motor function more than three levels
                            below the motor level on a given side)

Are at level half of the key muscles below the (single) neurological level graded 3 or better?
NO ↓   YES ↓
AIS=C   AIS=D

If sensation and motor function is normal in all segments, AIS=E
Note: AIS E is used in follow up testing when an individual with a documented SCI has recovered normal function. If an initial testing no deficits are found, the individual is neurologically intact; the ASIA Impairment Scale does not apply.

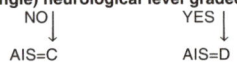

Fig. 5.15: ASIA scale.

F. Classification Spondylolisthesis

Wiltse, Neuman and Macnab's Classification

TABLE 5.6

Type		
I	Dysplastic	A: facet with axial orientation B: facet with sagittal orientation
II	Isthmic	A: lysis B: elongation C: fracture
III	Degenerative	
IV	Post-traumatic	
V	Pathologic	

Myerding Grading Spondylolisthesis

(Fig. 5.16 and Table 5.7)

TABLE 5.7

Grade I	25% of vertebral body has slipped forward
Grade II	50%
Grade III	75%
Grade IV	100%
Grade V	Vertebral body completely fallen off (i.e. spondyloptosis)

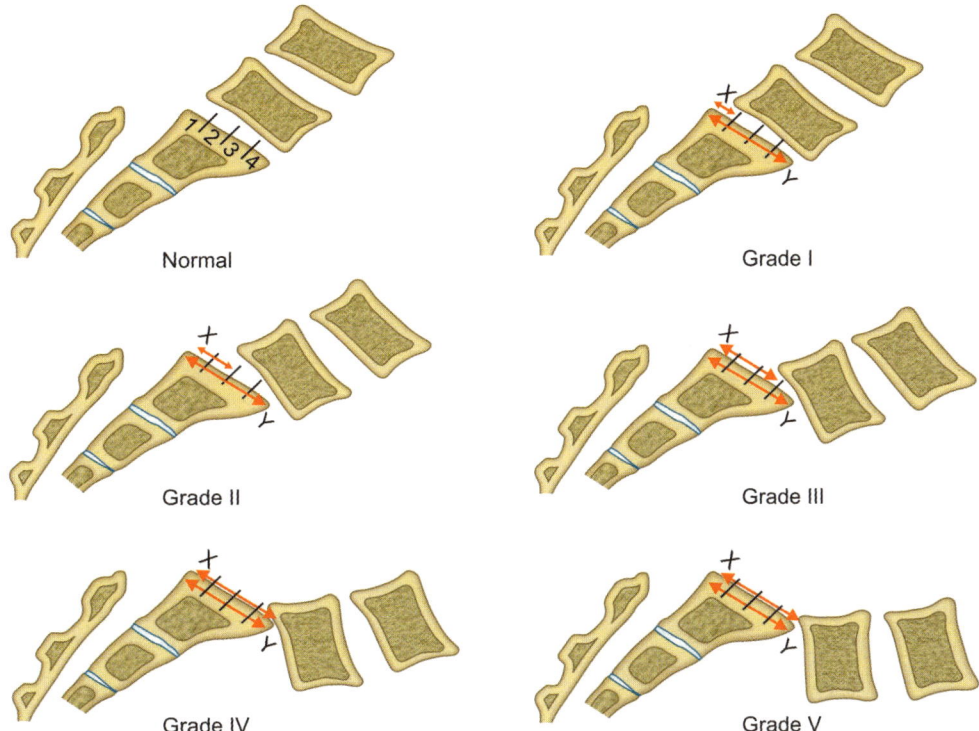

Fig. 5.16: Myerding grading spondylolisthesis depending on % of vertebral body slipped with respect to adjacent vertebrae.

5. SACRAL FRACTURES

Denis Classification (Fig. 5.17)

Zone 1. The region of the ala
- most common (50%)
- nerve injury rare (5%)
- usually occurs to L5 nerve root

Zone 2. The region of the sacral foramina
- may be stable/unstable
- zone 2 fracture with shear component highly unstable
- increased risk of nonunion and poor functional outcome

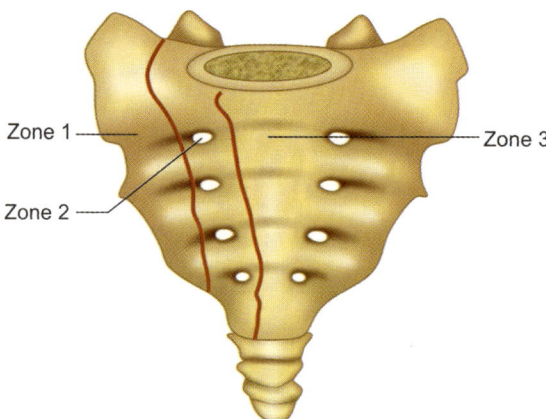

Fig. 5.17 Denis classification of sacral fractures.

Zone 3. The region of central sacral canal fracture medial to foramina into the spinal canal

- highest rate of neurologic deficit (60%)
- bowel, bladder, and sexual dysfunction

Transverse sacral fractures
- higher incidence of nerve dysfunction

U-type sacral fractures
- result's from axial loading
- represent: spino-pelvic dissociation
- high incidence of neurologic complications

6. TUBERCULOSIS SPINE

Kumar and Tuli's Staging of Potts Paraplegia

Stage 1. Patient unaware of neural deficit, physician detects plantar extensor and/or ankle clonus.

Stage II. Patient aware of deficit but manages to walk with support, clumsiness of gait.

Stage III. Paralysis in extension, sensory deficit less than 50%.

Stage IV. III + flexor spasm/paralysis in flexion/flaccid/sensory deficit more than 50%/sphincters involved.

Kumar's Clinicoradiological Classification (Tables 5.8 and 5.9)

TABLE 5.8

Stage		Features	Usual duration
I	Pre-destructive	Straightening, spasm, hyperemia	<3 months
II	Early-destructive	Diminished space paradiscal erosion Knuckle <10	2–4 months
III	Mild kyphos	2–3 verte k: 10–30	3–9 months
IV	Moderate kyphos	>3 verte K: 30–60	6–24 months
V	Severe kyphos	>3 verte K: >60	>2 years

TABLE 5.9

Stage	Clinicoradiological features	Usual duration
I. Pre-destructive	Straightening of curvatures, spasm of perivertebral muscles, scintiscan would show hyperemia	<3 months
II. Early destructive	Diminished disc space + paradiscal erosion (knuckle <10 degree) MRI shows marrow edema and break of osseous margins. CT-scan shows marginal erosion or cavitations	2–4 months
III, IV, V all have vertebral bodies destructive and collapse + appreciable kyphos		
III. Mild angular kyphos	2–3 vertebra involved (K: 10–30)	3–9 months
IV. Moderate angular kyphos	>3 vertebrae involved (K: 30–60)	6–24 months
V. Severe kyphos (Humpback)	>3 vertebrae involved (K > 60)	>2 years

K is the angle of kyphosis as measured by the technique of Dickson (1967). In stage III, IV, V, diagnosis is clear on conventional X-rays; CT scan and MRI would show advanced changes. However, these are unnecessary except for difficult sites (Kumar, 1988)

Seddon's Classification of Tuberculous Paraplegia

Group A (early onset paraplegia) a/k/a paraplegia associated with active disease:

- Active phase of the disease within first 2 years of onset.
- Pathology—inflammatory edema, granulation tissue, abscess, caseous material or ischemia of cord.

Group B (late onset paraplegia) a/k/a paraplegia associated with heated disease:

- After 2 years of onset of disease.
- Recrudescence of the disease or due to mechanical pressure on the cord.
- Pathology can be sequestra, debris, internal gibbus or stenosis of the canal.

7. SCOLIOSIS

TABLE 5.10: The Lenke classification system for AIS

Curve type	Proximal thoracic	Main thoracic	Thoracolumbar/lumbar	Description
1	Nonstructural	Structural*	Nonstructural	Main thoracic*
2	Structural*	Structural*	Nonstructural	Double thoracic
3	Nonstructural	Structural*	Structural×	Double major
4	Structural×	Structural§	Structural§	Triple major
5	Nonstructural	Nonstructural	Structural*	Thoracolumbar/lumbar (TL/L)
6	Nonstructural	Structural×	Structural*	Thoracolumbar/lumbar main thoracic (TL/L-MT)

*Major curve: largest Cobb measurement, always structural; ×Minor curve: remaining structural curve; §Type 4 – Mt or TL/L can be the major curve

Structural criteria (Minor curved)	
Proximal thoracic	• Side bending cobb = 25° • T2-T5 kyphosis = +20°
Main thoracic	• Side bending cobb = 25° • T10-L2 kyphosis = +20°
Thoracolumbar/lumbar	• Side bending cobb = 25° • T10-L2 kyphosis = +20°

Location of apex (SRS definition)	
Curve	Apex
Thoracic	T2 to T11-12 Disc
Thoracolumbar	T12-L1
Lumbar	L1-2 Disc to L4

Modifiers				
Lumbar spine modifier	Central sacral vertical line to lumber apex		Thoracic sagittal profile T5-T12 Modifier	Cobb angle
A	Between pedicles		– (Hypo)	<10°
B	Touches apical body (ies)		N (Normal)	10°–40°
C	Completely medial		+ (Hyper)	>40°

Curve Type (1–6) + Lumbar Spine Modifier (A, B, C) + Thoracic Sagittal Modifier (–, N, +) = Curve Classification (e.g. 1B+)

Chronological Classification Scoliosis

Divided into 3 subgroups based on the age onset:

- **Infantile** idopathic scoliosis (birth to 3 years old)
- **Juvenile** idiopathic scoliosis (4 to 10 years old)
- **Adolescent** idiopathic scoliosis (after 10 years old) → **the most common**

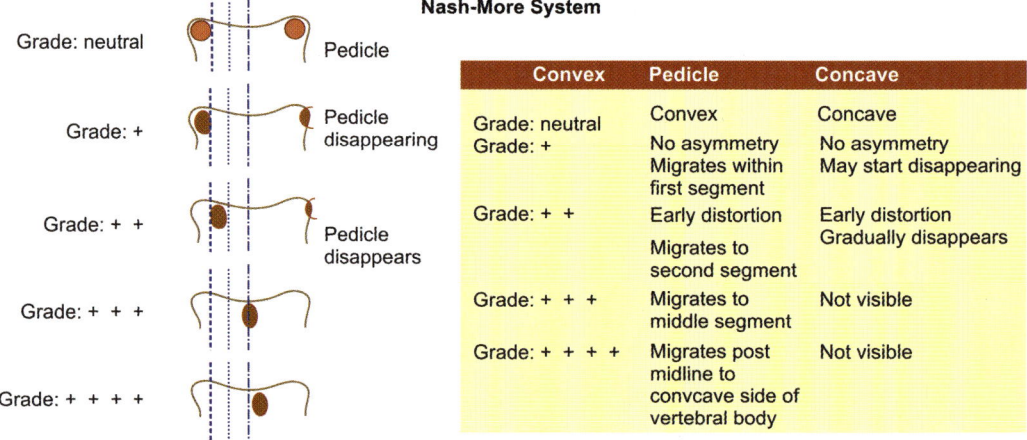

Fig. 5.18: Gradation of scoliosis according to Nash More system.

TABLE 5.11: King's classification scoliosis	
King type I: A S-shaped curve in which both the thoracic and lumbar curves cross the midline. The magnitude of the Cobb angle of the lumbar curve is larger than that of the thoracic curve on standing roentogenogram. Both curves are structural with nearly equal flexibility.	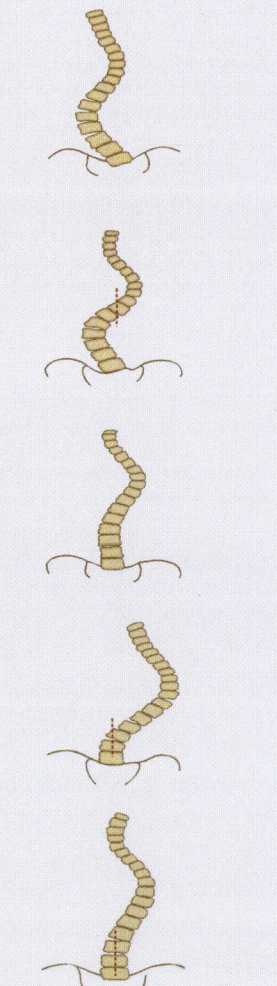
King type II: A S-shaped curve in which both the thoracic and lumbar curves cross the midline. The magnitude of the Cobb angle of the thoracic curve is larger than that of the lumbar curve on standing roentgenogram. The lumbar curve is more flexible.	
King type III: A thoracic curve in which the lumbar curve does not cross the midline (so called overhang).	
King type IV: A long thoracic curve in which L5 is centered over the sacrum, but L4 tilts into the long thoracic curve.	
King type V: A double thoracic curve with T1 tilted concavity of upper curve. The upper curve is structural on side bending.	

Risser Classification

The Risser classification (Fig. 5.19) is used to grade skeletal maturity based on the level of ossification and fusion of the iliac crest apophyses.

Stage 0. No ossification center at the level of iliac crest apophysis

Stage I. Apophysis under 25% of the iliac crest

Stage II. Apophysis over 25–50% of the iliac crest

Stage III. Apophysis over 50–75% of the iliac crest

Stage IV. Apophysis over >75% of the iliac crest

Stage V. Complete ossification and fusion of the iliac crest apophysis.

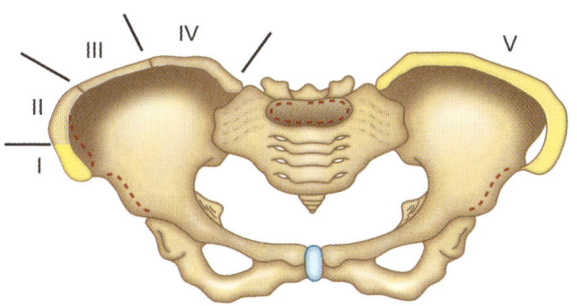

Fig. 5.19: Risser sign

Sprengel Shoulder

Cavendish Classification

Grade I (Very mild): Shoulders level; deformity invisible when patient is dressed.

Grade II (Mild): Shoulders almost level; deformity visible as a lump in the web of the neck when patient is dressed.

Grade III (Moderate): Shoulder joint is elevated 2–5 centimeters; deformity visible.

Grade IV (Severe): Shoulder joint is elevated; superior angle of the scapula near the occiput.

Radiographic Rigault's Classification (Fig. 5.20)

The Rigault's classification is used to radiographically classify the extent of superior positioning of the scapula based on the relationship of the superomedial angle of the scapula to the spine.

Grade 1 (mild) deformity occurs when the superomedial angle of the scapula lies between the second and fourth thoracic transverse processes (TP).

Grade 2 (moderate) deformity occurs when it lies between the fifth cervical and second thoracic TP.

Grade 3 (severe) deformity occurs when it lies above the fifth cervical TP.

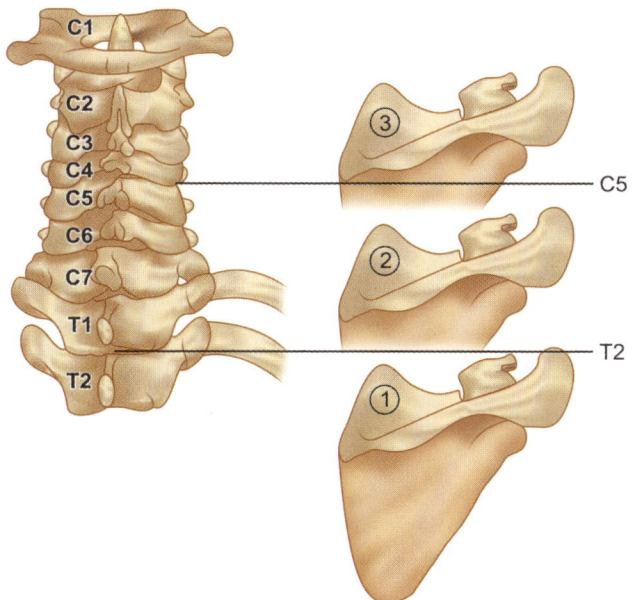

- **Grade 1:** Superomedial angle lower than T2 but above T4 transverse process

- **Grade 2:** Superomedial angle located between C5 and T2 transverse process

- **Grade 3:** Superomedial angle above C5 transverse process

Fig. 5.20: Rigault's classification.

Pediatric Injuries

GENERAL TERMS

Plastic Deformation

Immature bone is weaker in bending strength but absorbs more energy before fracture. This is a result of the ability of immature bone to undergo plastic (permanent) deformation. Although plastic deformation has been described in adults, it is much more common in children. Plastic deformation is most common in the forearm (Fig. 6.1), particularly the ulna, especially after isolated radial head dislocation; however, it has been noted in the femur as well.

Although bone in young children may re-model after plastic deformation, most authors recommend reduction of plastic deformation of the forearm if there is more than 20 degrees of angulation or the child is older than 4 years and has a clinically evident deformity or limitation of pronation and supination.

Buckle (Torus) Fractures

Buckle fractures, also called torus fractures because of their resemblance to the base of an architectural column, most commonly occur at the transition between the metaphyseal woven bone and lamellar bone of the diaphyseal cortex. Buckle fractures represent a spectrum of injuries from mild plastic deformation of one area of the cortex to complete fractures with a buckled appearance (Fig. 6.2).

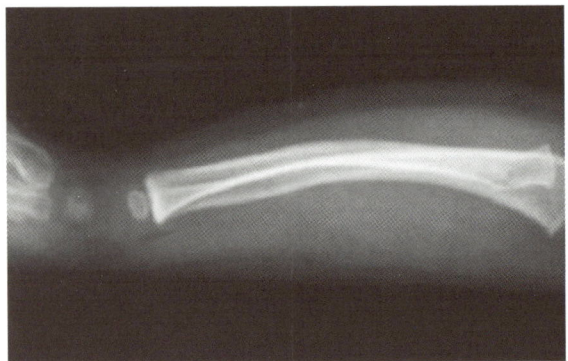

Fig. 6.1: Plastic deformity—see the angulation without any break. *Source*: Reproduced from Chee Y (2009). Plastic deformity. EURORAD. DOI:10.1594/EURORAD/CASE.2791.

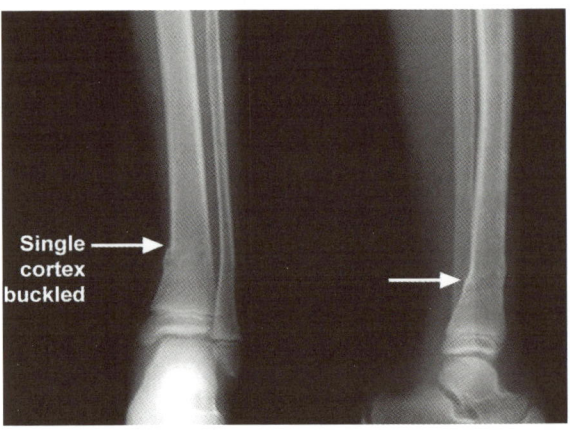

Single cortex buckled

Fig. 6.2: X-ray leg AP and lateral views showing torus fracture of distal tibial metaphysis.

Greenstick Fractures (Fig. 6.3)

Greenstick fractures are unique to children because immature bone is more flexible and has a thicker periosteum than mature adult bone. In a greenstick fracture, the cortex in tension fractures completely whereas the cortex and periosteum in compression remain intact but frequently undergo plastic deformation. It has been said that it is necessary to complete the fracture on the intact compression side of greenstick fractures.

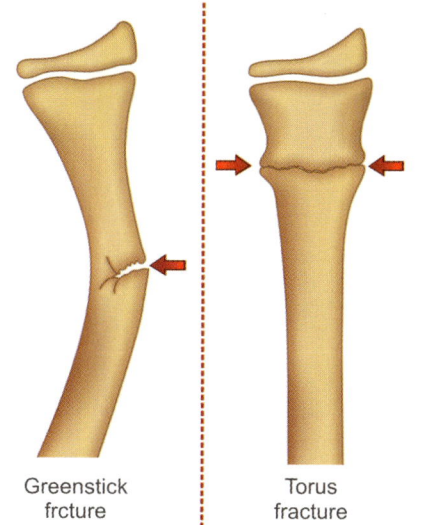

Greenstick frcture   Torus fracture

Fig. 6.3: Comparision between greenstick fracture and torus fracture.

1. PEDIATRIC PHYSEAL INJURY CLASSIFICATION

- Poland
- Aitkens (1936)
- Salter and Harris (1963)
- Ogden (1981)
- Peterson (1994)

A. Poland (1898)

Consisted of four types of physeal fractures. Types I, II, and III were the foundation of the Salter-Harris classification (Fig. 6.4).

Poland type I. Epiphyseal separation without metaphyseal fragment, or extension into the epiphysis.

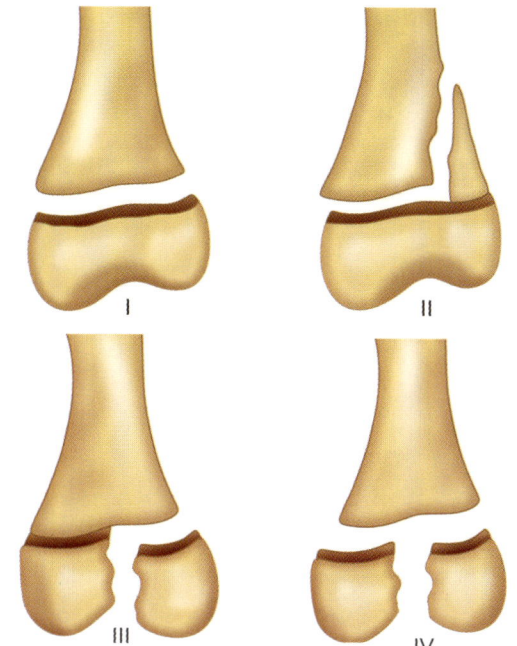

Fig. 6.4: Poland classification of physeal injury.

Poland type II. Physeal fracture line extends into the metaphysis.

Poland type III. Fracture extends from the articular surface to the physis and continues peripherally through the physis.

Poland type IV. T-condylar fracture of the epiphysis and physis.

B. Aitkens (1936) (Fig. 6.5)

Type I. Corresponded to Poland and Salter-Harris type II fractures.

Type II. Poland and Salter-Harris type III fractures.

Type III. An intra-articular transphyseal metaphyseal-epiphyseal fracture equivalent to a Salter-Harris type IV fracture.

C. Salter-Harris Classification (Figs 6.6 to 6.8)

Salter and Harris published their commonly used five-part classification of physeal injuries in 1963. The first four types were adopted from Poland (types I, II, and III) and Aitken (Aitken type III became Salter-Harris type IV). Salter

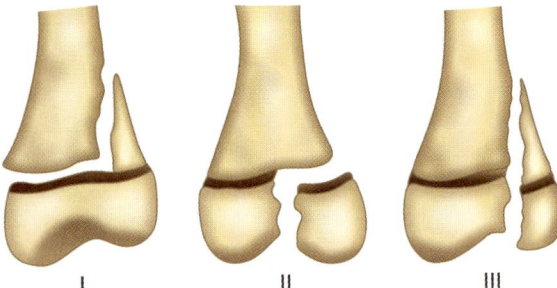

Fig. 6.5: Aitkens classification.

and Harris added a fifth type, which they postulated was an unrecognized compression injury characterized by normal X-rays and late physeal closure.

Type I. Transphyseal fracture involving the hypertophic and calcified zones; prognosis is usually excellent, although complete or partial growth arrest may occur in displaced fractures.

Type II. Transphyseal fracture that exits the metaphysis; the metaphyseal fragment is known as the Thurston-Holland fragment; the periosteal hinge is intact on the side with the metaphyseal fragment; prognosis is excellent, although complete or partial growth arrest may occur in displaced fractures (Fig. 6.6).

Type III. Transphyseal fracture that exits the epiphysis, causing intra-articular disruption; anatomic reduction and fixation without violating the physis are essential; prognosis is guarded because partial growth arrest and resultant angular deformity are common problems.

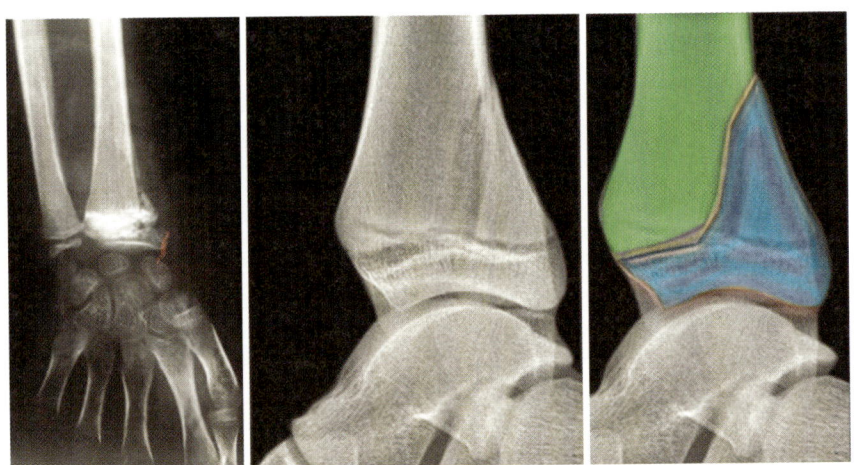

Fig. 6.6: Salter-Harris type II fracture showing Thurston-Holland fragment.

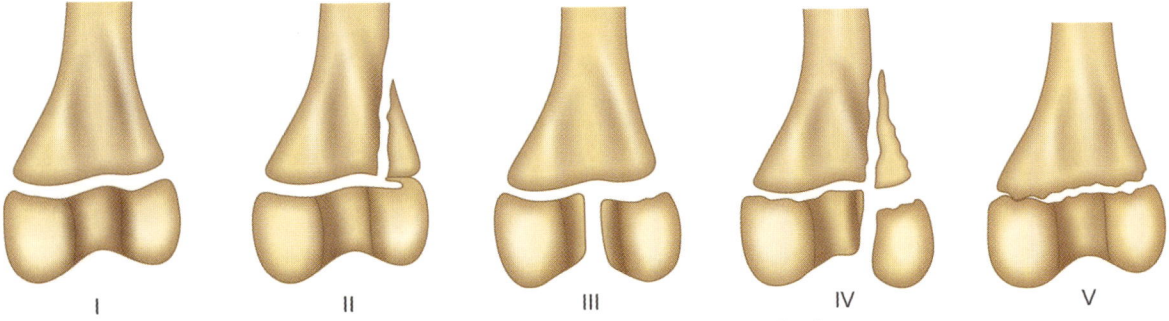

Fig. 6.7: Salter-Harris classification of physeal (growth plate) injuries.

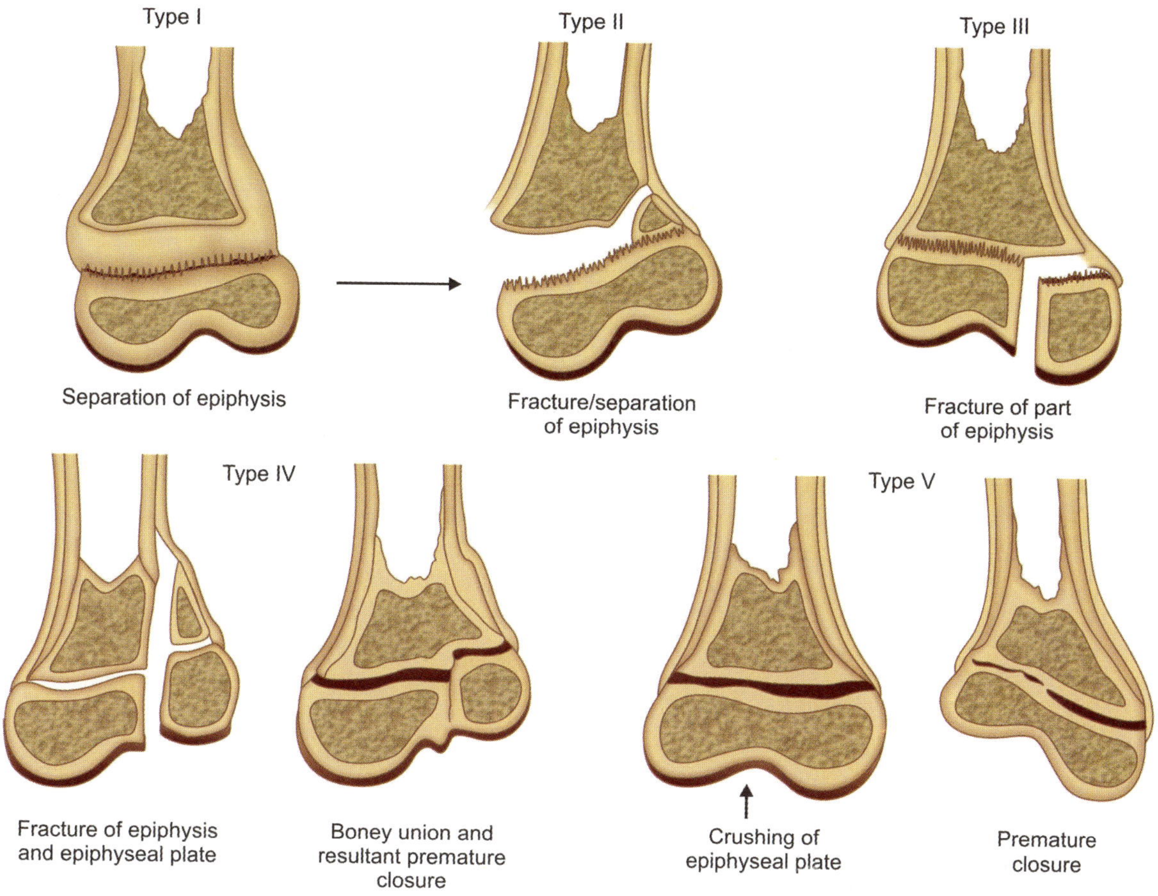

Type I

Type II

Type III

Separation of epiphysis

Fracture/separation
of epiphysis

Fracture of part
of epiphysis

Type IV

Type V

Fracture of epiphysis
and epiphyseal plate

Boney union and
resultant premature
closure

Crushing of
epiphyseal plate

Premature
closure

Fig. 6.8: Salter-Harris physeal fracture classification showing relationship with growth plate.

Type IV. Fracture that traverses the epiphysis and the physis, exiting the metaphysis; anatomic reduction and fixation without violating the physis are essential; prognosis is guarded, because partial growth arrest and resultant angular deformity are common.

Type V. Crush injury to the physis; diagnosis is generally made retrospectively; prognosis is poor because growth arrest and partial physeal closure commonly result.

Type VI. (Rang on 1969) Bruise or contusion to periphery of the epiphyseal plate. It can cause scaring, tethering and arrest of the periphery of the epiphyseal plate, producing angular deformity. It is also included in ogden system of classification (Fig. 6.9).

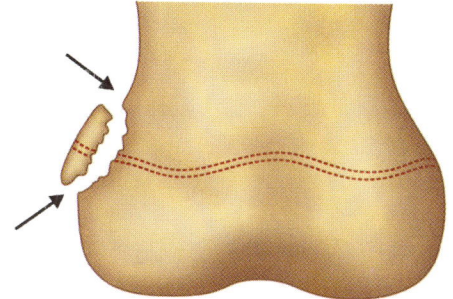

Fig. 6.9: Salter-Harris type VI published by Rang

Ogden type VII. Fracture involving the epiphysis only, osteochondral fracture and epiphysis avulsion.

Ogden type VIII. Metaphyseal fracture. Primary circulation to the remodelling region of the cartilage cell columns is disrupted. Hypervascularity may cause angular deformities.

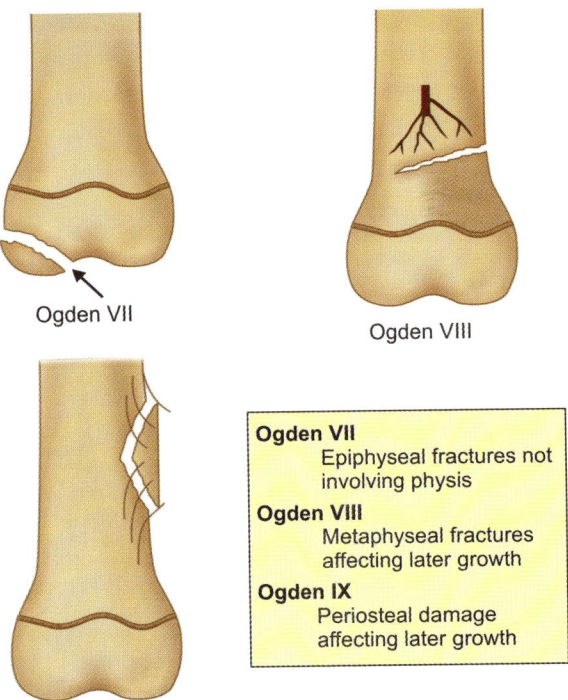

Ogden VII

Ogden VIII

Ogden VII
Epiphyseal fractures not involving physis

Ogden VIII
Metaphyseal fractures affecting later growth

Ogden IX
Periosteal damage affecting later growth

Ogden IX

Fig. 6.10: Pictorial representation of Ogden physeal fracture types.

Ogden type IX. Diaphyseal fracture. The mechanism for appositional growth (the periosteum) is interrupted. Prognosis is good, if, reduction maintained. Cross union between radius/ulna and tibia/fibula can occur if intermingling of periosteum takes place.

D. Peterson (1994)

Peterson based on his epidemiological study of 951 fractures proposed a new classification system (Fig. 6.11) challenging the existence of Salter Harris type V, as he didn't find this type in any of his samples. His classification retained Salter-Harris types I through IV as Peterson types II, III, IV, and V and added two new types. It is important to be cognizant of the two new patterns that Peterson described, because they are clinically relevant.

Peterson's type I. Transverse metaphyseal fracture with a longitudinal extension to the physis It is subclassified into four types, based on the extent of metaphyseal comminution and fracture pattern. Sites-distal radius and finger phalanx.

Peterson's type VI. Partial physeal loss. Unfortunately, this pattern of injury currently is common, largely as a consequence of lawnmower injuries. Soft tissue loss, neurovascular injury, and partial physeal loss (usually including the epiphysis so that articular impairment also results) further complicate this often-devastating injury.

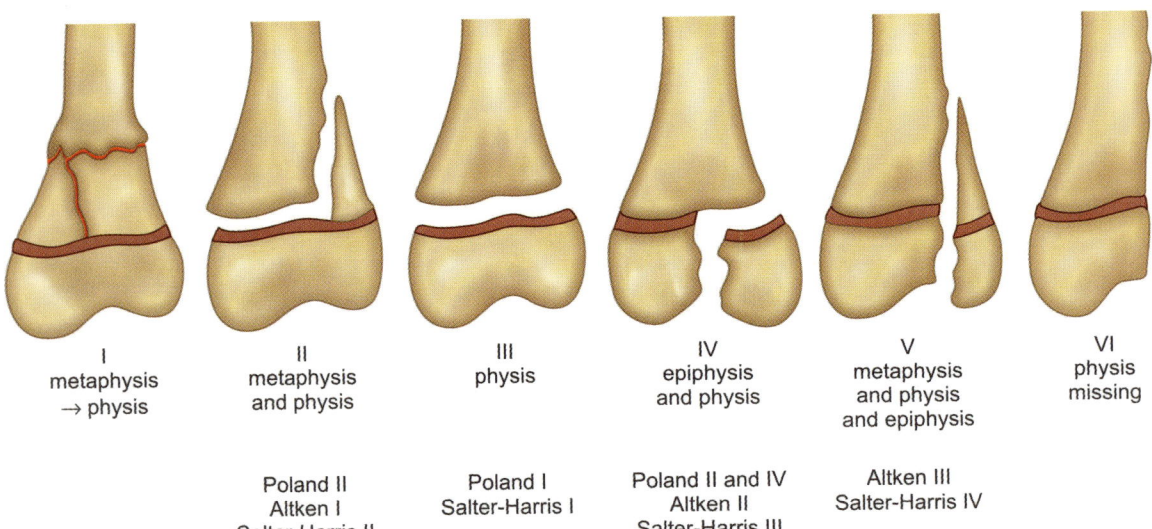

I metaphysis → physis	II metaphysis and physis	III physis	IV epiphysis and physis	V metaphysis and physis and epiphysis	VI physis missing
	Poland II Altken I Salter-Harris II	Poland I Salter-Harris I	Poland II and IV Altken II Salter-Harris III	Altken III Salter-Harris IV	

Fig. 6.11: Peterson physeal fracture classification system.

2. SUPRACONDYLAR HUMERUS FRACTURES

A. Classification of Extension Type

Gartland Classification (Figs 6.12 and 6.13)

Based on degree of displacement:

Type I. Nondisplaced. The anterior cortex is broken and the posterior cortex remains intact and there is no or minimal angulation at the fracture site.

Type II. Displaced with intact posterior cortex; may be slightly angulated or rotated

Type III. Complete displacement; postero-medial or posterolateral

Type IV. New addition. Displaces into extension and flexion, i.e both periosteum is injured. Mainly diagnosed with manipulation under C-arm.

B. Wilkins Modification of Gartland's Classification

Extension Type

Type 1. Undisplaced

Type 2.
- *Type 2A.* Intact posterior cortex and angulation only
- *Type 2B.* Intact posterior cortex, angulation and rotation

Type 3
- *Type 3A.* Completely displaced, no cortical contact, posteromedial

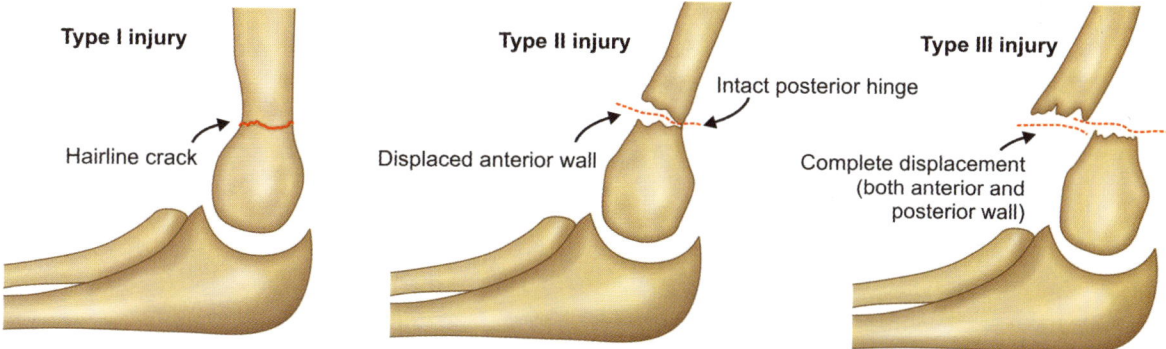

Fig. 6.12: Pictorial representation of Gartland classification of supracondylar fracture of humerus.

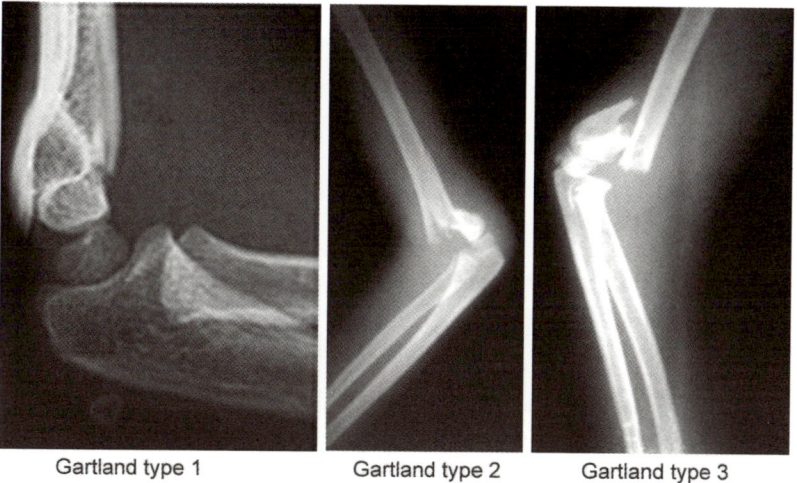

Fig. 6.13: X-ray representation of Gartland's classification of supracondylar fracture of humerus.

- *Type 3B.* Completely displaced, no cortical contact, posterolateral.

Flexion Type Fracture

Type I. Undisplaced

Type II. Displaced with intact anterior cortex.

Type III. Complete displacement, antero-laterally.

C. AO Classification

With regard to the degree of displacement at four levels.

Type I. No displacement.

Type II. Displacement in one plane.

Type III. Rotation of the distal fragment with displacement in two planes.

Type IV. Rotation with displacement in three planes, i.e. no contact between bone fragments.

3. LATERAL CONDYLAR PHYSEAL FRACTURES

A. Milch Classification (Fig. 6.14)

Type I. Fracture line courses lateral to the trochlea and into the capitelotrochlear groove, representing a Salter-Harris type IV fracture. The elbow is stable because the trochlea is intact. They are Salter Harris type IV fracture.

Type II. Fracture line extends into the apex of the trochlea, representing a Salter-Harris type II fracture. The elbow is unstable because the trochlea is disrupted. Type II fracture are unstable and may allow for radio-ulnar translocation if capsuloligamentous disruption occurs on the contralateral side.

B. Jakob et al Classification (Fig. 6.15)

- *Stage I.* Undisplaced with intact articular surface (Badelon modification – displacement <2 mm).
- *Stage II.* Complete fracture through articular surface.

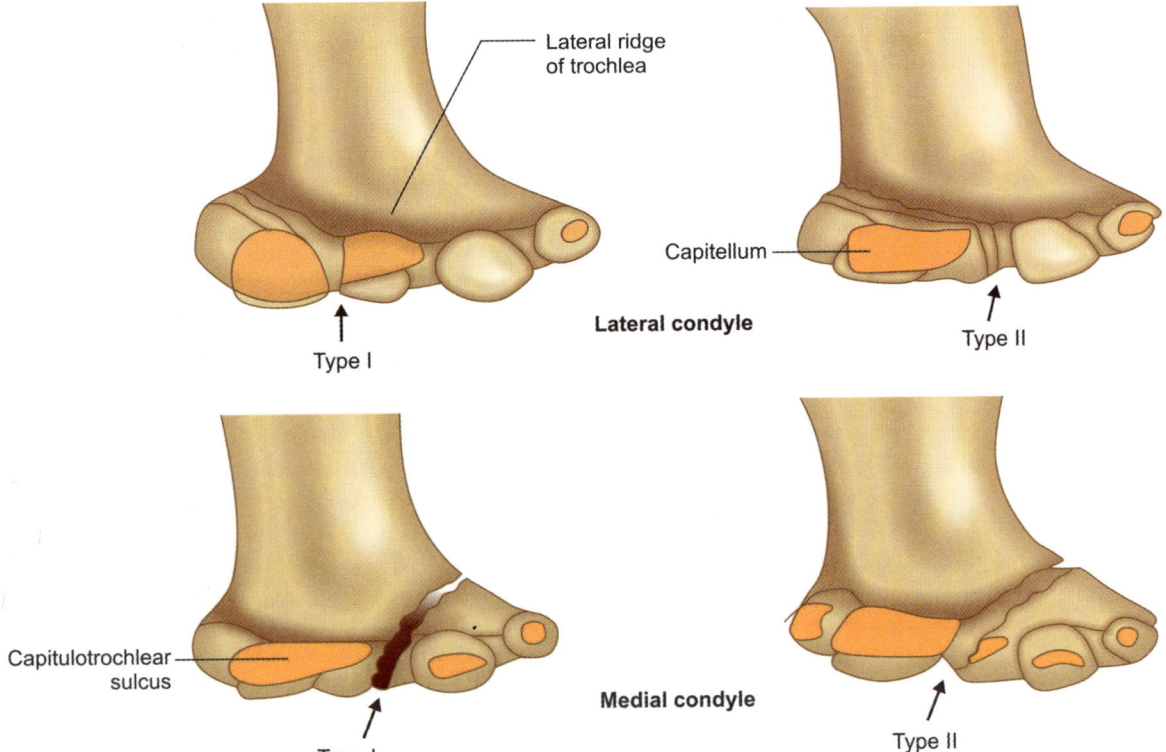

Fig. 6.14: Milch classification of lateral condyle humerus physeal fractures.

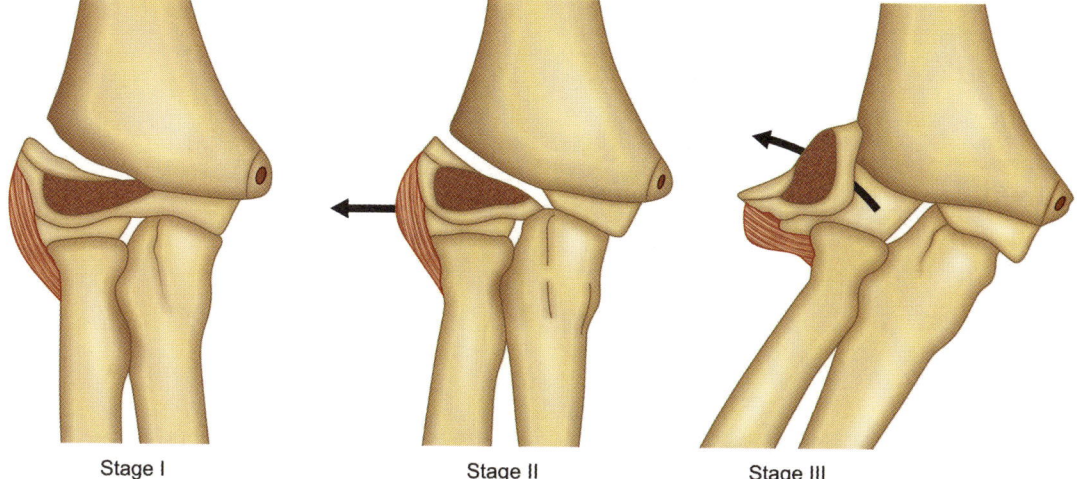

Stage I   Stage II   Stage III

Fig. 6.15: Jakob et al classification of lateral condyle humerus fracture.

- *Stage III.* Fragment rotated, displaced laterally and proximally allowing translocation of olecranon and radial head.

Finnbogason and associates classification: They classified only minimally displaced fractures, i.e. ≤2 mm.
- *Type A.* Minimal/no gap on radial side/dorsal side. # not continuous to epiphyseal cartilage.
- *Type B.* As above but # line continuous to articular surface.
  Lateral # gap > medial.
- *Type C.* As of B but # gap as wide medially as laterally.

Weiss et al
- *Type I.* <2 mm displacement
- *Type II.* >2 m displacement

- *Type III.* >2 mm displacement but no intact articular surface.

4. MEDIAL CONDYLAR PHYSEAL FRACTURES

Kilfoyle Classification (Fig. 6.16)

Type I. Impacted or greenstick fracture, i.e. nondisplaced, articular surface intact.

Type II. A fracture through the humeral condyle into the joint (i.e. fracture lne complete) with little or no displacement.

Type III. An epiphyseal fracture that is intra-articular and involves the medial condyle with the fragment displaced and rotated due to pull by flexor mass.

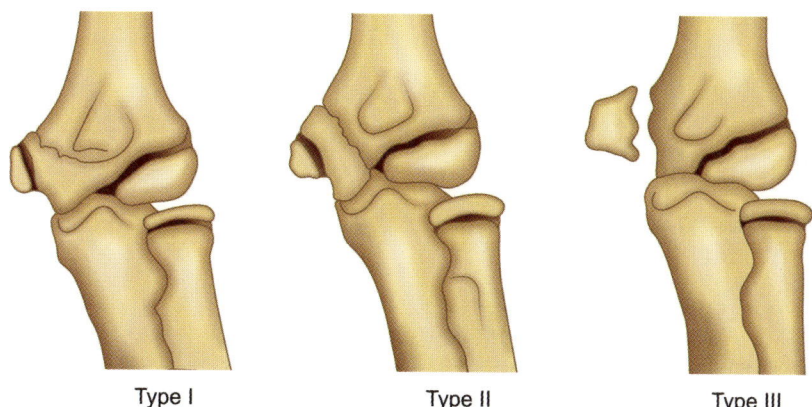

Type I   Type II   Type III

Fig. 6.16: Kilfoyle classification of medial condyle humerus fracture.

5. TRANSPHYSEAL FRACTURES

Delee Classification

Based on ossification of the lateral condyle:

Group A. Infant, before appearance of lateral condylar ossification center (birth to 7 months of age); diagnosis easily missed; Salter-Harris type I.

Group B. Lateral condyle ossified (7 months to 3 years); Salter-Harris type I or II (fleck of metaphysis).

Group C. Large metaphyseal fragment, usually exiting laterally (ages 3 to 7 years).

6. T-CONDYLAR FRACTURES

Wilkins and Beaty Classification

Type I. Nondisplaced or minimally displaced.

Type II. Displaced, with no metaphyseal comminution.

Type III. Displaced, with metaphyseal comminution.

7. RADIAL HEAD AND NECK FRACTURES

A. Wilkins Classification (Fig. 6.17)

Based on meachanism of injury.

Type A. Salter-Harris type I or II physeal injury.

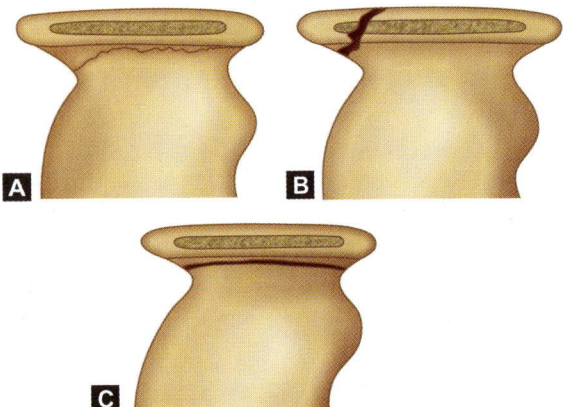

Fig. 6.17: Wilkins classification of pediatric radial head and neck fractures.

Type B. Salter-Harris type III or IV intra-articular injury.

Type C. Fracture line completely within metaphysic.

Type D. Fractures occurring when a dislocated elbow is being reduced.

Type E. Fracture occurring with elbow dislocation.

- Fracture associated with elbow dislocation
  - Reduction injury
  - Dislocation injury.

B. O'Brien Classification (Fig. 6.18)

Based on degree of angulation of the superior articular surface from the horizontal.

Type I. <30°

Type II. 30–60°

Type III. >60°

8. MONTEGGIA'S FRACTURE

Fracture of the shaft of the ulna with associated dislocation of the proximal radio ulnar joint.

A. Bado Classification (Fig. 6.19)

The classification is based on mechanism of injury and does not deal with treatment/ prognosis.

Type I. Anterior dislocation of the radial head with fracture of the ulnar diaphysis at any level with anterior angulation.

Type II. Posterior/posterolateral dislocation of the radial head with fracture of the ulnar diaphysis with posteriorangulation.

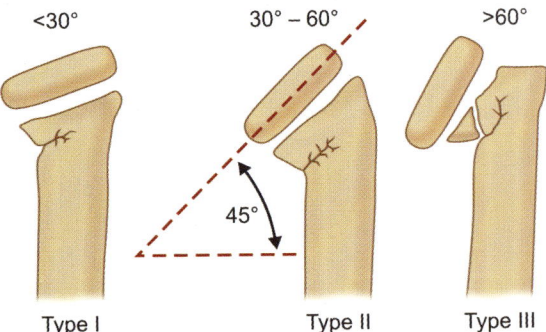

Fig. 6.18: O'Brien classification.

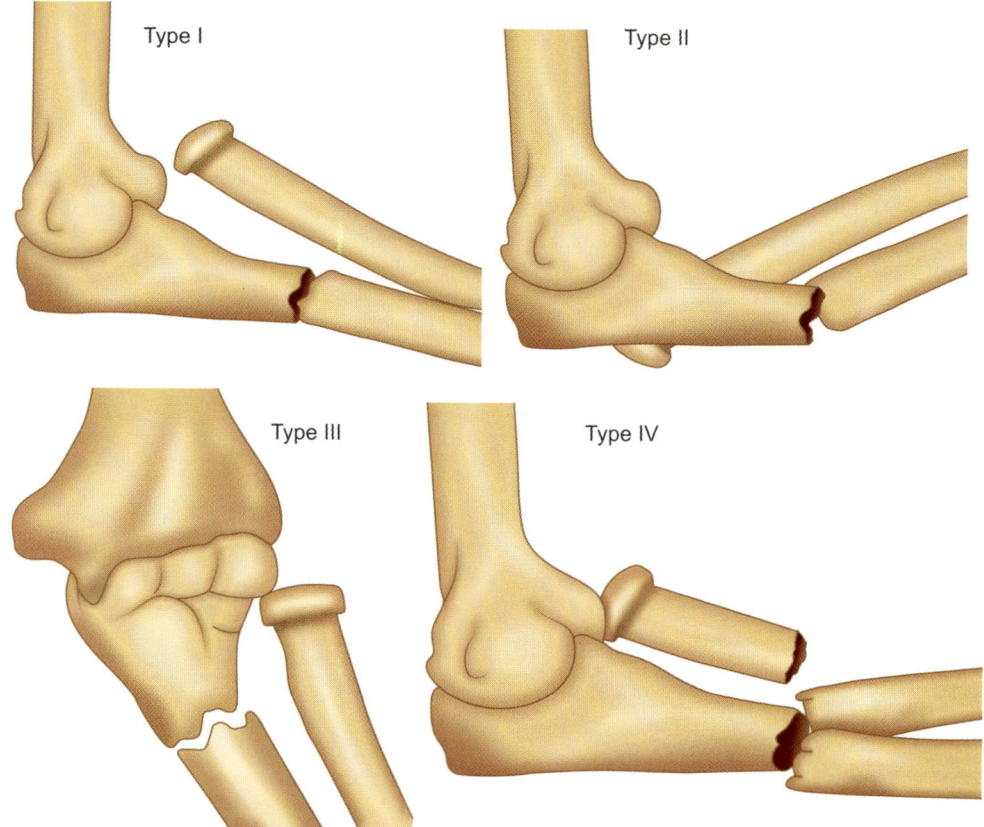

Fig. 6.19: Bado classification.

Type III. Lateral/anterolateral dislocation of the radial head with fracture of the ulnar metaphysis. This occurs almost exclusively in children, but isolated cases in adults have been described.

Type IV. Anterior dislocation of the radial head with fractures of both the radius and ulna within proximal third at the same level. This occurs almost exclusively in adult patients.

B. Jupiter et al Further Subdivided Bado Type II

IIA. Ulnar # involving coronoid process and olecranon.

IIB. # distal to coronoid at the junction of metaphysis—diaphysis.

IIC. Ulnar # strictly diaphyseal.

IID. Complex pattern of ulna # from olecranon to ulna diaphysis.

C. Letts Classification of Monteggia's Fracture Dislocation (Fig. 6.20)

Dislocation of the radial head with fracture of ulna

A. Anterior dislocation of the radial head with plastic deformation of the ulna.

B. Anterior dislocation of the radial head with greenstick fracture of ulna.

C. Anterior dislocation of the radial head with complete fracture of ulna.

D. Posterior dislocation of the radial head with fracture of ulnar metaphysic.

E. Lateral dislocation of the radial head with metaphyseal greenstick fracture of the ulna.

D. Monteggia Equivalents

Type I

• Isolated dislocation of radial head.

• Radial neck fracture (isolated).

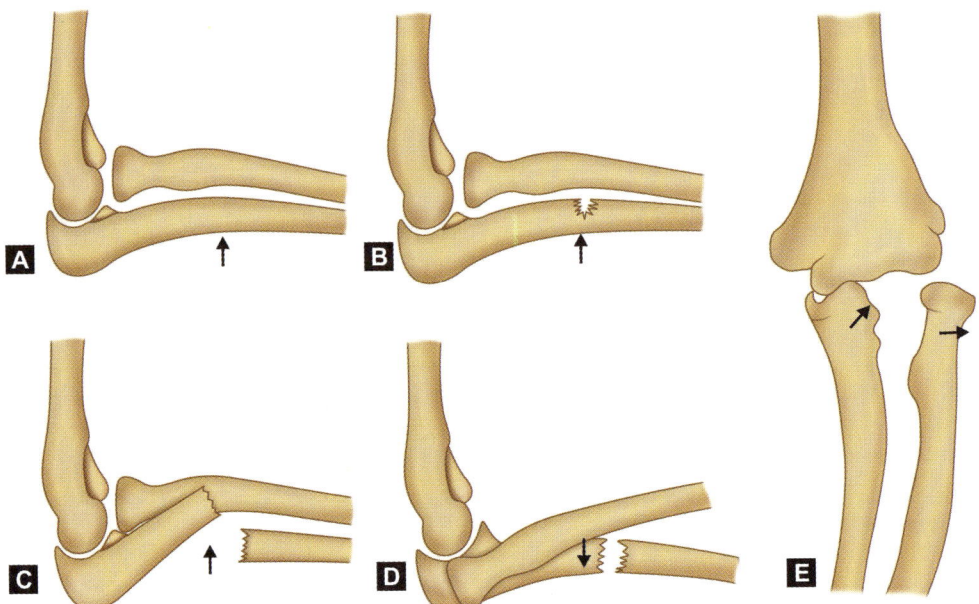

Fig. 6.20: Lets clasification of Monteggia's fractures.

- Radial neck fracture in combination with a fracture of the ulnar diaphysis.
- Radial and ulnar fractures with the radial fracture above the junction of the middle and proximal thirds.
- Fracture of ulnar diaphysis with anterior displocation of radial head and an olecranon fracture.

Type II
- Posterior dislocation of the elbow
- Posterior dislocation of radial head associated with fracture of radial epiphysis/neck.

Type III. Described by **Ravessoud**
- An oblique fracture of the ulna with varus alignment and a displaced lateral condylar fracture.

Type IV. Described by **Arazi**.
- Fracture of the distal humerus with ulnar diaphysis fracture and fracture of radial neck.

Galeazzi Fracture: Rare in Children
Fracture of the radial shaft with dislocation of the distal radioulnar joint. They are sub-classified according to the distance of the radial fracture from the articular surface.

Type I. Occur within 7.5 cm of the articular surface of the distal radius.
- Ulnar head anteriorly dislocated more commonly.

Type II. They occur proximally
- Ulnar head posteriorly dislocated.

Variant: In children separation of DRUJ occurs through a displaced Salter Harris type II physeal fracture of distal ulna. However, in adult DRUJ dislocation cannot occur without disruption of the triangular fibrocartilagenous complex, but in children with open physis, the distal ulnar physis can avulse before rupture of the complex and interposition of the periosteum may block rotation.

9. SCAPHOID

Classification
Type A. Fractures of the distal pole
- *Type A1.* Extra-articular distal pole fractures
- *Type A2.* Intra-articular distal pole fractures.

Type B. Fractures of the middle third.

Type C. Fractures of the proximal pole.

10. VINCE AND MILLER SYNOSTOSIS

According to Location

Type I. Intra-articular fracture in the distal 1/3rd.

Type II. Nonarticular in the distal/middle 1/3rd after severe trauma.

Type III. Synostosis in the proximal 1/3rd. It may occur even after mild injury, non-operative treatment and severe trauma.

Risk of synostosis increases by surgical trauma to the soft tissue between radius, ulna and excision of radial head alone is a greater risk than open reduction is.

However, Vince and Miller didnot discuss rationale for their grading.

PEDIATRIC LOWER LIMB FRACTURE CLASSIFICATION

11. PELVIC FRACTURE

A. Young and Burgess Classification
(Fig. 6.21)

a. Lateral Compression Force

Type I. The posterolateral force results in a sacral and pubic ramus fracture.

Type II. The anterolateral force results in an additional iliac wing fracture.

Type III. Further force creates an opening injury to the contralateral pelvis with disruption of the sacrospinous, sacrotuberous, and anterior sacroiliac ligaments.

Anteroposterior compression (APC)

Lateral compression (LC)

Vertical shear (VS)

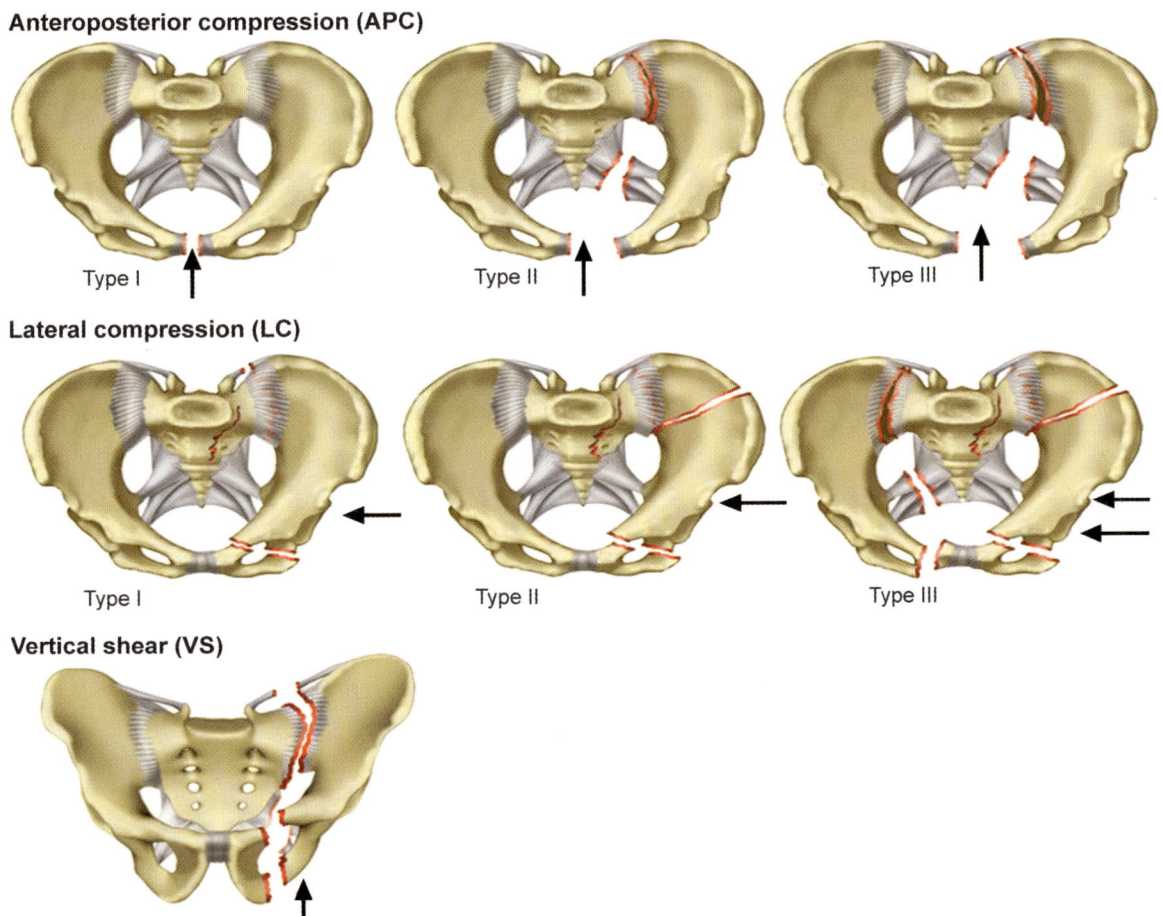

Fig. 6.21: The Young and Burgess classification of pelvic fractures. Arrows show the direction of force.

b. Anteroposterior Compression Force

Type I. Disruption of the symphysis pubis.

Type II. Disruption of the anterior ligaments.

Type III. Disruption of the posterior ligaments.

c. Vertically Directed Force

Creating fractures in the rami and disruption of the sacrospinous joint.

B. Tile Classification

Not used often in pediatric fractures.

C. Torode and Zieg Classification (Fig. 6.22)

Type I. Avulsion fractures.

Type II. Iliac wing fractures.

Type III. Simple pelvic ring fractures.

Type IV. Pelvic ring disruption fractures.

12. ACETABULUM

Acetabular fractures in children are best classified into four types:

Type I. Small fragment fractures that occur with dislocation of the hip.

Type II. Linear fractures that result in one or more large, stable fragments.

Type III. Linear fractures that result in hip instability.

Type IV. Fractures that are secondary to central dislocations of the hip.

13. HIP DISLOCATION

Stewart-Milford Classification

Most commonly used classification for hip fracture-dislocations.

Grade I. No acetabular fracture or only a minor chip fracture.

Grade II. Posterior rim fracture but with hip stability after reduction.

Grade III. Posterior rim fracture with hip instability after reduction.

Grade IV. Dislocation accompanied by fracture of the femoral head.

14. DELBET CLASSIFICATION OF PEDIATRIC HIP FRACTURES (Fig. 6.23)

Type I. Transepiphyseal fracture, anatomically they are similar to salter-Harris type I fracture. High chances of AVN. Closest D/D is SCFE.

Type II. Transcervical fracture, most common type.

Type III. Cervicotrochanteric fracture.

Type IV. Pertrochanteric/intertrochanteric fracture.

15. TIBIAL SPINE (INTERCONDYLAR EMINENCE) FRACTURES

Meyers and Mckeever Classification (Fig. 6.24)

Type I. Minimal or no displacement of fragment.

Type II. Angular elevation of anterior portion with intact posterior hinge.

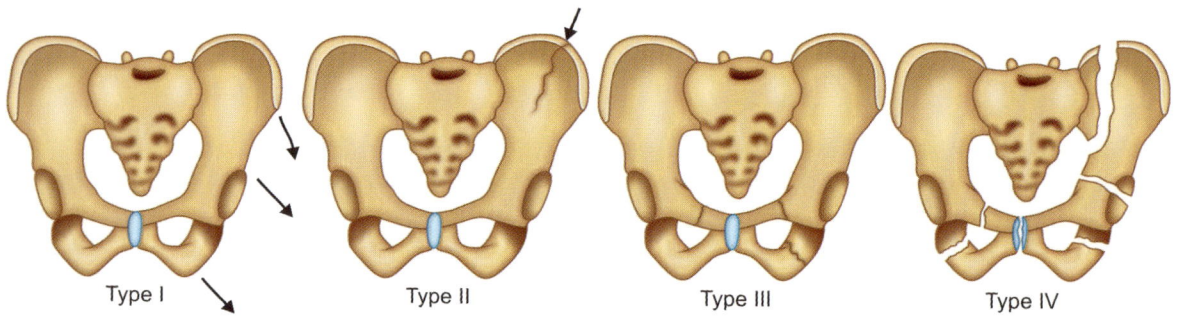

| Type I | Type II | Type III | Type IV |

Fig. 6.22: Torode and Zieg classification.

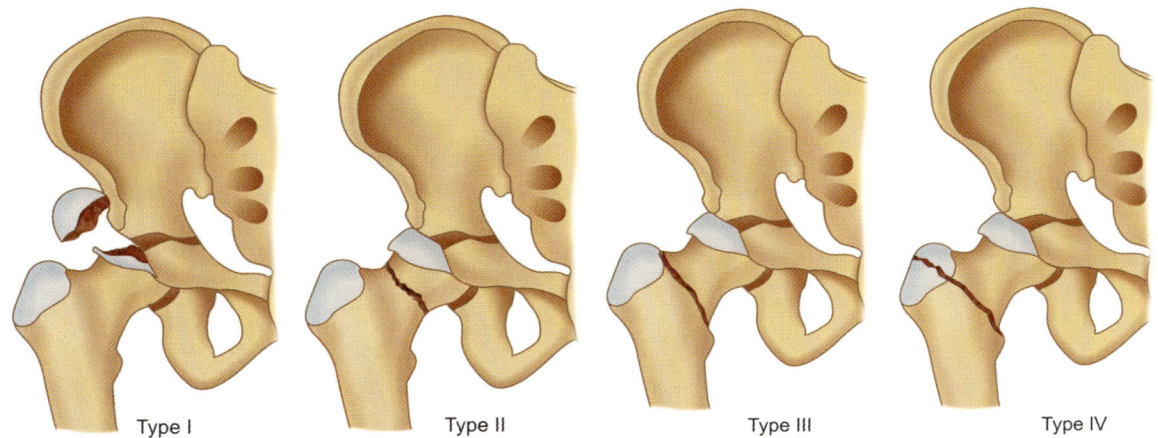

Fig. 6.23: Delbet classification of pediatric hip fractures.

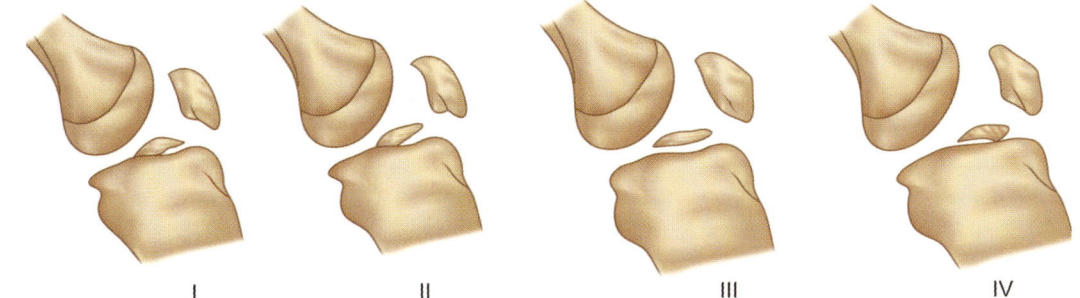

Fig. 6.24: Meyers and Mckeever classification.

Type III. Complete displacement with or without rotation.

Zaricznyj added a type IV fracture, where the fragments are comminuted.

16. TIBIAL TUBEROSITY FRACTURE

Normal tibia/tibial tubercle epiphysis—its important to know how normal tibia/tibial tubercle physis looks like (Fig. 6.25) to understand its injury classification.

Watson-Jones Classification (Fig. 6.26)

OGDEN modified the classification types I, II, III into type I, II, III A and B each to account for degree of displacement and comminution.

Type I. A small fragment, displaced superiorly
- *Type IA.* Injuries are minimally displaced
- *Type IB.* Injuries are hinged anteriorly and proximally.

Type II. A larger fragment involving the secondary center of ossification and proximal tibial epiphysis
- *Type IIA.* Injuries are simple fractures and
- *Type IIB.* Injuries are comminuted.

Type III. A fracture that passes proximally and posteriorly across the epiphyseal plate and proximal articular surface of tibia (Salter-Harris type III)
- *Type IIIA.* Complete tubercle fracture without comminution
- *Type IIIB.* Complete tubercle fracture with comminution.

Ryes and Deberham added type IV. Anterior tubercle fracture line extends completely across the tibial physis in a Salter-Harris type I pattern.
- *Type IVA.* Strictly physeal injury.
- *Type IVB.* Posterior metaphyseal fragment, consistent with Salter-Harris type II.

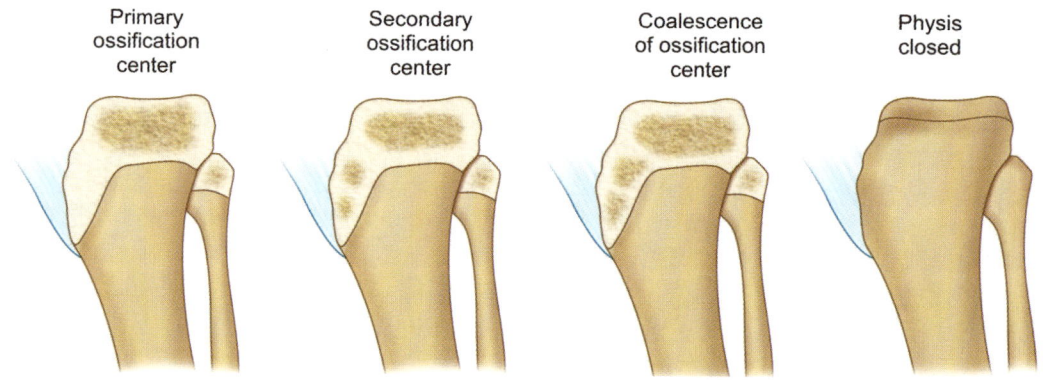

Fig. 6.25: Normal tibia/tibial tubercle physis.

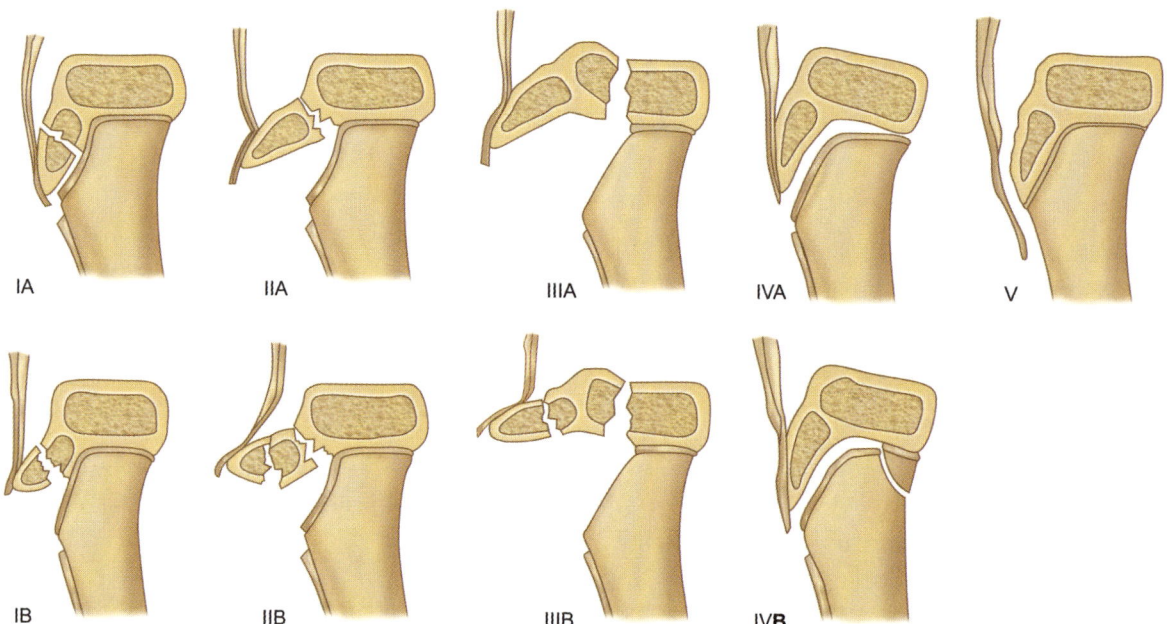

Fig. 6.26: Watson-Jones classification of tibial tuberosity fracture with Ogden modification and, Ryes and Deberham and Curtis and Mccoy addition.

Curtis and Mccoy et al type V. Salter-Harris type III extension and an associated type IV fracture giving the fracture a 'Y' configuration.

17. ANKLE FRACTURE

Dias and Tachdjian modified the Lauge-Hansen classification to include the Salter-Harris classification so that it applies to injuries in children. The original classification defined four types of fractures (Figs 6.27 to 6.30), each with a two-part name; the first term refers to the position of the foot at the time of injury and the second term to the direction of the deforming force, with grades of injury described in increasing severity. Subsequently, the last four types of fractures were added: juvenile Tillaux, triplane, axial compression, and miscellaneous.

Tillaux fracture (Fig. 6.31) results from external rotation of the ankle and occurs as a result of asymmetric closure of the distal tibial physis. Closure of the distal tibial physis

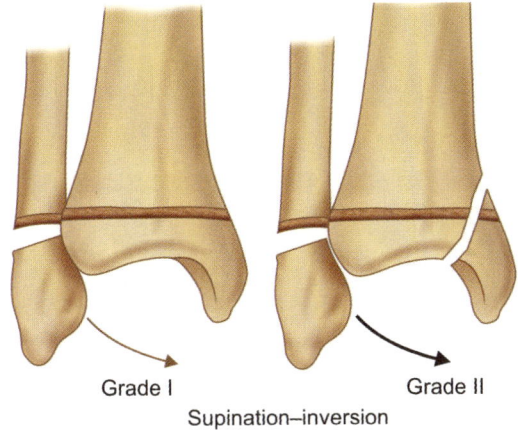

Grade I   Grade II

Supination–inversion

Fig. 6.27: Supination and inversion type of ankle injury with different grades.

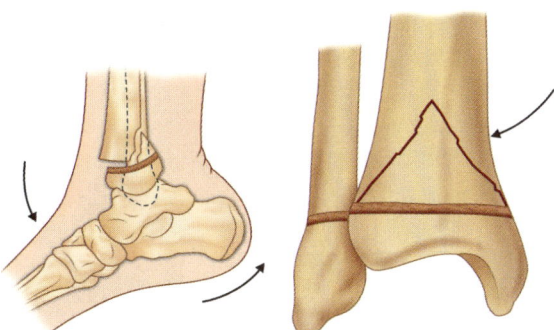

Fig. 6.28: Supination and plantar flexion type of ankle injury.

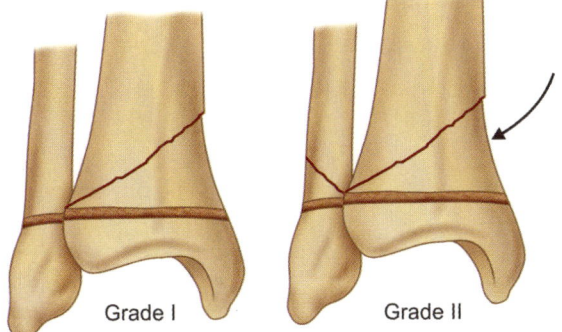

Grade I   Grade II

Fig. 6.29: Supnation–external rotation type of injury.

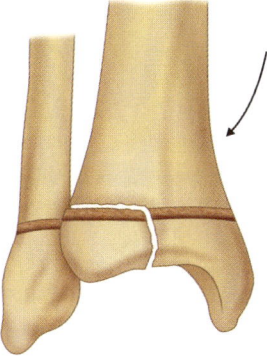

Fig. 6.30: Pronation–eversion–external rotation type of ankle injury.

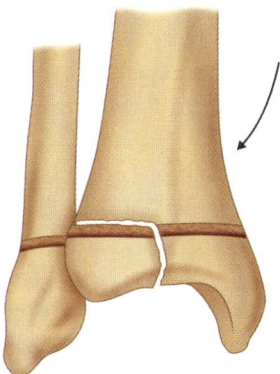

Fig. 6.31: Tillaux fracture.

begins centrally followed by medial closure (13–14 years of age) and ultimately lateral closure (14.5–16 years of age). It is during this 18-month window that patients are pre-disposed to this particular fracture. When the distal lateral physis is still open and an external rotation force is applied to the foot, an avulsion fracture of the anterolateral distal epiphysis occurs as the inferior tibiofibular ligament pulls this fragment free. This is a Salter-Harris type III fracture with a vertical fracture line that extends from the articular surface proximally, through the lateral physis, and out the lateral cortex. In an older child the fracture line occurs more laterally because the physis has closed medially. The fracture fragment and the amount of displacement tend to be less in this age group, although this is variable.

Triplane fracture (Fig. 6.32). The fracture is so named because the fracture lines occur in three planes. The injury is thought to be an external rotation force applied to a supinated foot. The coronal fracture line begins in the physis and

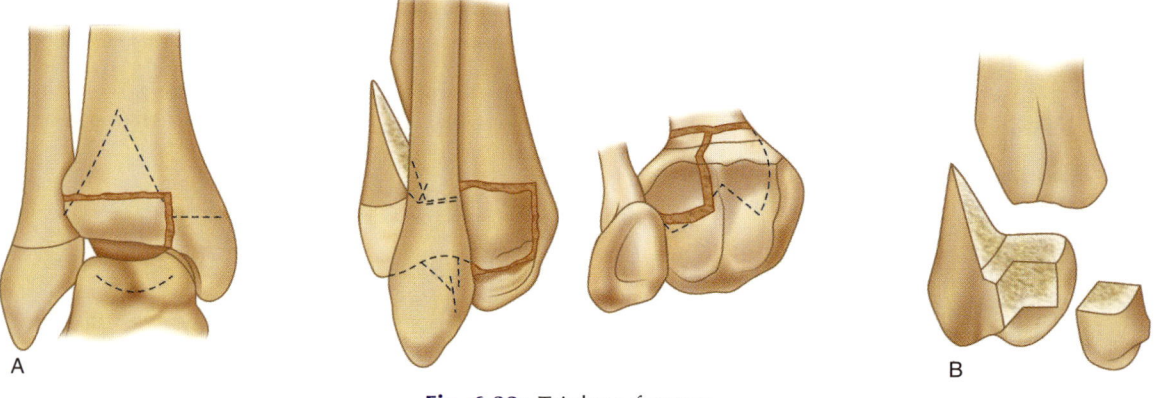

A   B

Fig. 6.32: Triplane fracture.

travels proximally through the posterior metaphysis; the sagittal fracture travels from the midjoint line to the physis and results in an anteromedial and often an anterolateral fragment; and the transverse fracture travels digitorum longus through the physis. These fracture lines can result in either a two-part or a three-part triplane fracture.

Hawkins Classification (Fig. 6.33)

This fractures was first described by Hawkins in 1970. His three-part classification was primarily based on the amount of fracture displacement and provided information on the prognosis for AVN. This classification was

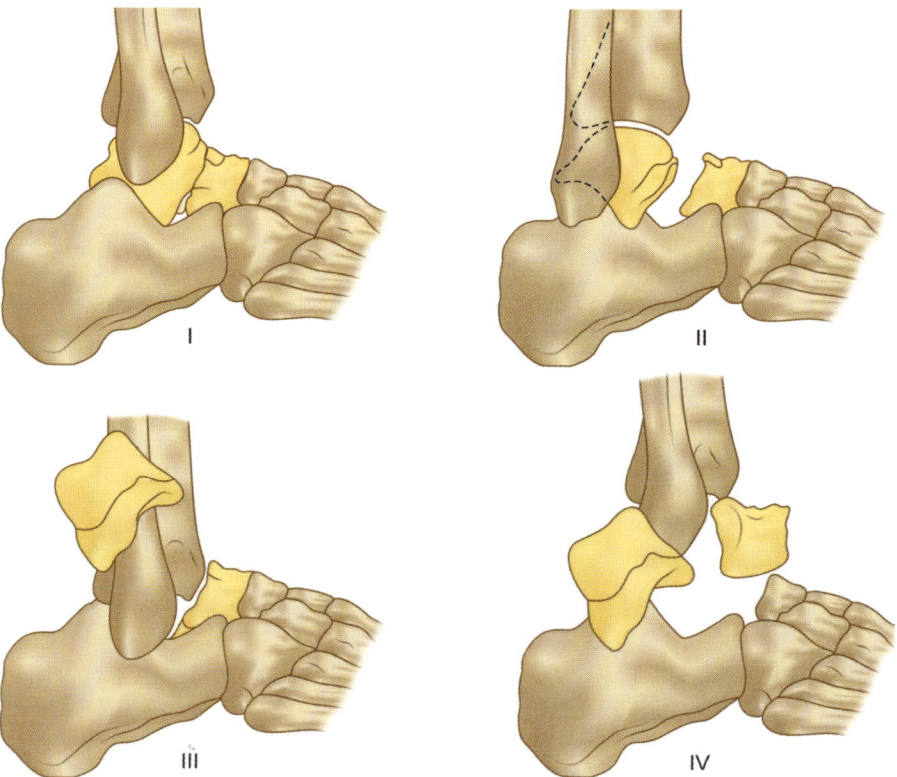

I   II

III   IV

Fig. 6.33: Hawkins classification of talus fracture.

later modified by Canale and Kelly to include a fourth type.

Type I. Injury is an undisplaced vertical fracture of the talar neck.

Type II. Fracture is a displaced fracture; the subtalar joint is subluxated or dislocated but the ankle joint is normal.

Type III. Injury is similar to a type II injury, but subluxation or dislocation of both the ankle and subtalar joints occurs.

Type IV. Injury is very rare and is characterized by dislocation of the talar head from the talonavicular joint.

19. CALCANEAL FRACTURE: SCHMIDT AND WEINER (Fig. 6.34)

Type 1
- *A.* Fracture of the tuberosity or apophysis
- *B.* Fracture of the sustentaculum tali
- *C.* Fracture of the anterior process
- *D.* Distal inferolateral fracture
- *E.* Small avulsion of the body.

Type 2. Fracture of the posterior and/or superior parts of the tuberosity.
- *A.* Beak fracture
- *B.* Avulsion fracture of the insertion of the Achilles tendon.

Type 3. Linear fracture of the body not involving the subtalar joint.

Type 4. Non displaced or minimally displaced linear fracture of the body involving the subtalar joint.

Type 5. Compression fracture through the subtalar joint.

- *A.* Tongue type
- *B.* Joint depression type.

Type 6. Any fracture with significant soft tissue injury, bone loss, and loss of insertion of the Achilles tendon.

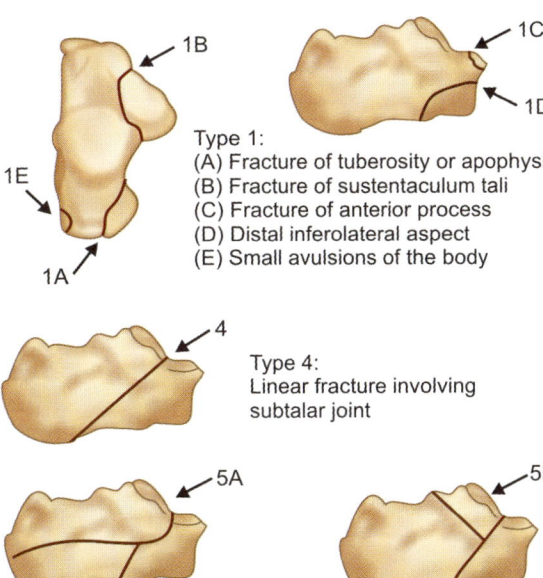

Type 1:
(A) Fracture of tuberosity or apophysis
(B) Fracture of sustentaculum tali
(C) Fracture of anterior process
(D) Distal inferolateral aspect
(E) Small avulsions of the body

Type 4:
Linear fracture involving subtalar joint

Type 5: Compression fracture of subtalar joint
(A) Tongue type; (B) Joint-depression type

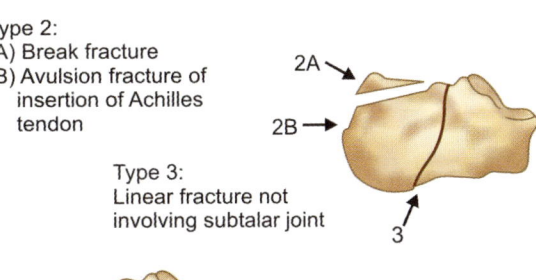

Type 2:
(A) Break fracture
(B) Avulsion fracture of insertion of Achilles tendon

Type 3:
Linear fracture not involving subtalar joint

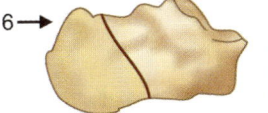

Type 6:
Significant bone loss of posterior aspect with loss of Achilles tendon insertion

Fig. 6.34: Schmidt and Weiner classification of calcaneal fracture.

Periprosthetic Fractures

PERIPROSTHETIC HIP FRACTURES AFTER THR

1. FEMUR

A. INTRAOPERATIVE FRACTURE (Fig. 7.1): VANCOUVER CLASSIFICATION

The Vancouver classification of periprosthetic femoral fractures has been altered to include intraoperative fractures and perforations.

Type A. Fractures are confined to the proximal metaphysis.

Type B. Fractures involve the proximal diaphysis but can be treated with long stem fixation.

Type C. Fractures extend beyond the longest revision stem and may include the distal femoral metaphysis.
   Each type is subdivided into:
* Simple perforations (subtype 1),
* Nondisplaced(subtype 2), or
* Displaced (subtype 3).

B. VANCOUVER CLASSIFICATION (DUNCAN AND MASRI) (Fig. 7.2)

Duncan and Masri proposed a classification system for postoperative periprosthetic femoral fractures.

Type A. Involve the trochanteric area (AG involve the greater trochanter, AL involve the lesser trochanter).

Type B. Fractures around the stem or extending slightly distal to it.
* B1 implant well fixed,
* B2 implant loose, bone stock adequate,
* B3 implant loose, bone stock inadequate due to osteolysis, osteoporosis, and fracture comminution.

Type C. Fractures distal to the stem that the presence of the femoral component may be ignored.

C. JOHANSSON CLASSIFICATION

Type I. Fracture proximal to prosthetic tip with the stem remaining in the medullary canal.

Type II. Fracture extending beyond distal stem with dislodgement of the stem from the distal canal.

Type III. Fracture entirely distal to the tip of the prosthesis.

D. COOKE AND NEWMAN (MODIFICATION OF BETHEA) (Fig. 7.3)

Type I. Explosion type with comminution around the stem; the prosthesis is always loose, and the fracture is inherently unstable.

Type II. Oblique fracture around the stem; fracture pattern is stable, but prosthetic loosening usually is present.

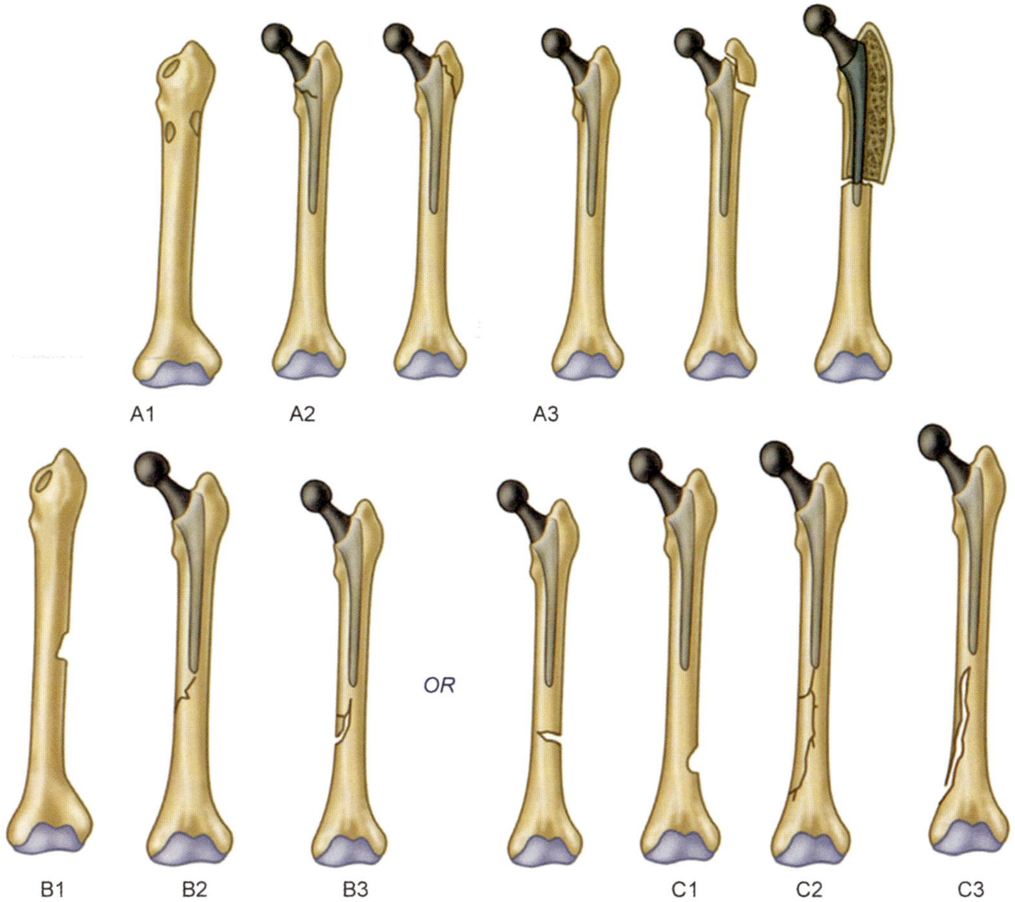

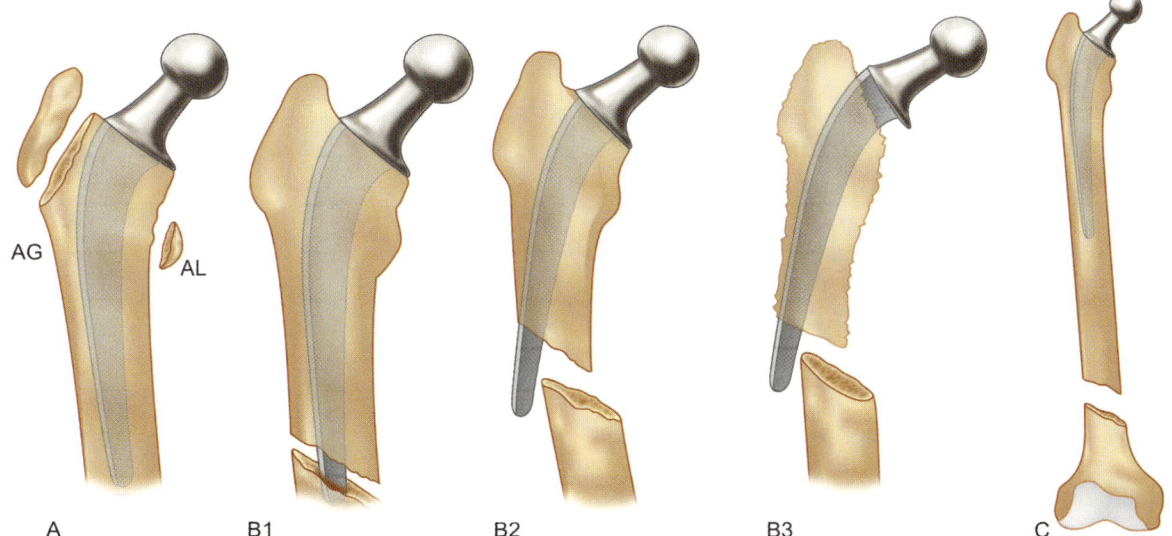

Fig. 7.1: Intraoperative periprosthetic fractures of femur.

A1   A2   A3

B1   B2   B3   OR   C1   C2   C3

AG   AL

A   B1   B2   B3   C

Fig. 7.2: Vancouver classification (Duncan and Masri) periprosthetic femoral fractures.

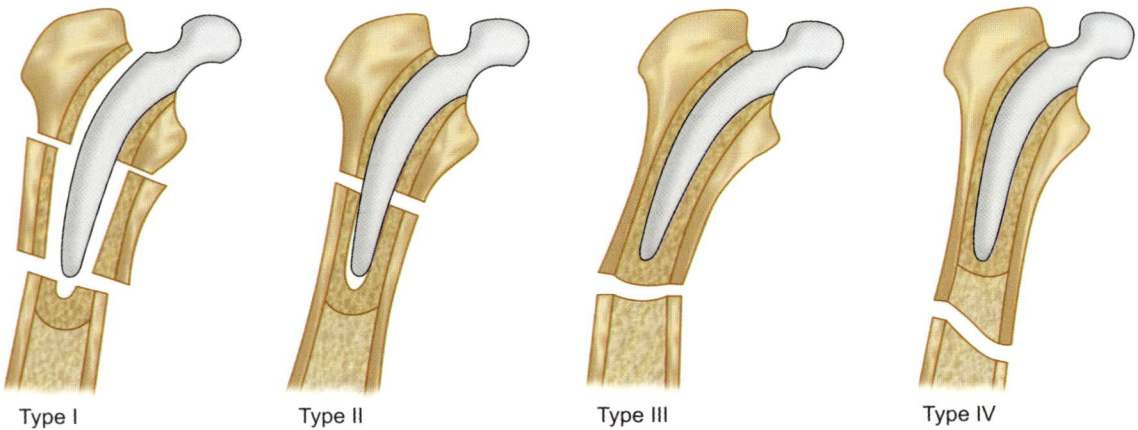

| Type I | Type II | Type III | Type IV |

Fig. 7.3: Cooke and Newman classification of periprosthetic femoral fractures.

Type III. Transverse fracture at the distal tip of the stem; the fracture is unstable, but prosthetic fixation is usually unaffected.

Type IV. Fracture entirely distal to prosthesis; fracture is unstable, but prosthetic fixation is usually unaffected.

2. ACETABULUM

DAVIDSON et al CLASSIFICATION

Davidson et al. described a periprosthetic acetabular fracture classification based on the extent of the fracture and stability of the implant.

Type I. Fractures are nondisplaced and the cup is stable.

Type II. Fractures are nondisplaced but with potential instability due to the fracture pattern, such as a transverse or posterior column fracture.

Type III. Injuries are significantly displaced and inherently unstable.

PERIPROSTHETIC KNEE FRACTURES AFTER TKR

FEMORAL FRACTURES

1. LEWIS AND RORABECK CLASSIFICATION (Fig. 7.4)

Type I. Undisplaced fractures, prosthesis intact.

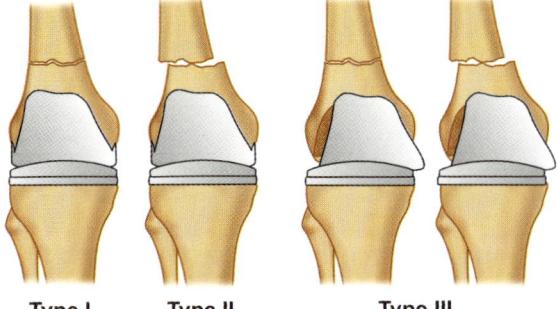

| Type I | Type II | Type III |

Fig. 7.4: Lewis and Rorabeck classification of periprosthetic femoral fracture in total knee replacement.

Type II. Displaced fractures, prosthesis intact.

Type III. Displaced or undisplaced fracture, prosthesis loose or failing.

2. NEER CLASSIFICATION, WITH MODIFICATION BY MERKEL (Fig. 7.5)

Type I. Minimally displaced supracondylar fracture.

Type II. Displaced supracondylar fracture.

Type III. Comminuted supracondylar fracture.

Type IV. Fracture at the tip of the prosthetic femoral stem of the diaphysis above the prosthesis.

Type V. Any fracture of the tibia.

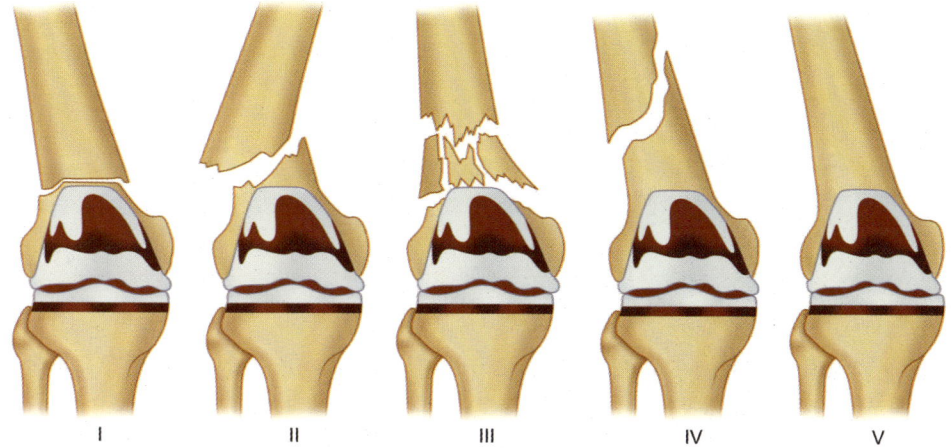

Fig. 7.5: Neer's periprosthetic fracture of the knee.

TIBIAL FRACTURES (NEER AND MERKEL TYPE V)

1. GOLDBERG CLASSIFICATION

Type I. Fractures not involving cement/implant composite or quadriceps mechanism.

Type II. Fractures involving cement/implant composite and/or quadriceps mechanism.

Type III
- *Type IIIA.* Inferior pole fractures with patellar ligament disruption.
- *Type IIIB.* Inferior pole fractures without patellar ligament disruption.

Type IV. Fracture dislocation.

2. CLASSIFICATION FOR PERIPROSTHETIC FRACTURES OF THE TIBIA ASSOCIATED WITH TOTAL KNEE ARTHROPLASTY (TKA)

There are four types Felix, Stuart and Hansen (Fig. 7.6):

Type I. Fracture involves the tibial plateau.

Type II. Fracture is adjacent to the prosthetic stem.

Type III. Fracture is distal to the stem.

Type IV. Fracture involves the tibial tubercle.

Subclassified as:
A—prosthesis radiographically well fixed,
B—loose, and
C—intraoperative.

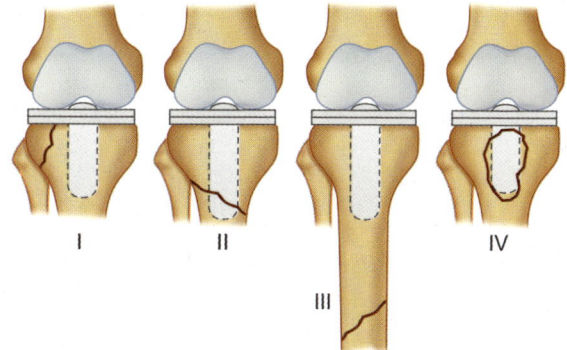

Fig. 7.6: Periprosthetic tibia fracture in total knee replacement.

Periprosthetic Patella Fracture in TKA

Type I. Fractures associated with an intact extensor mechanism and stable implant.

Type II. Displaced fractures with extensor mechanism discontinuity.

Type III. Loose patellar component.

PERIPROSTHETIC SHOULDER FRACTURES

1. UNIVERSITY OF TEXAS AT SAN ANTONIO CLASSIFICATION (Fig. 7.7)

Type I. Fractures occurring proximal to the tip of the humeral prosthesis.

Type II. Fractures occurring in the proximal portion of the humerus with distal extension beyond the tip of the humeral prosthesis.

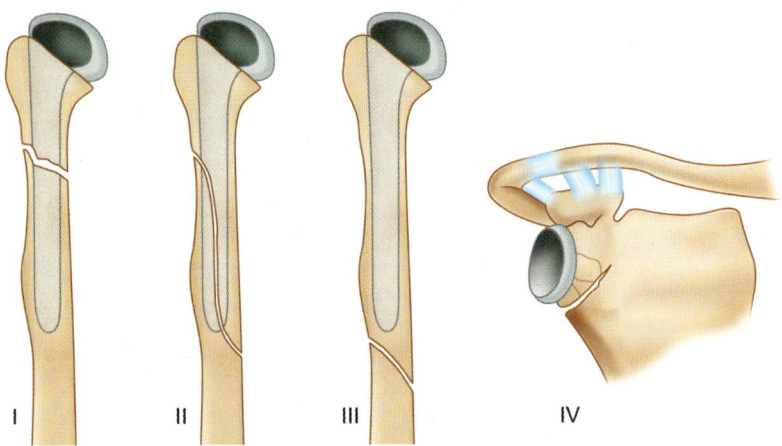

Fig. 7.7: Periprosthetic shoulder fractures.

Type III. Fractures occurring entirely distal to the tip of the humeral prosthesis.

Type IV. Fractures occurring adjacent to the glenoid prosthesis.

2. WRIGHT AND COFIELD

Humerus fracture after total shoulder arthroplasty (Fig. 7.8).

Wright and Cofield classified periprosthetic humeral shaft fractures into three types.

Type A. Centered at the tip of the stem and extending proximally more than one-third of the length of the stem.

Type B. Centered at the tip of the stem with less proximal extension.

Type C. Involving the distal humeral diaphysis, distal to the tip of the stem, and extending into the metaphysic.

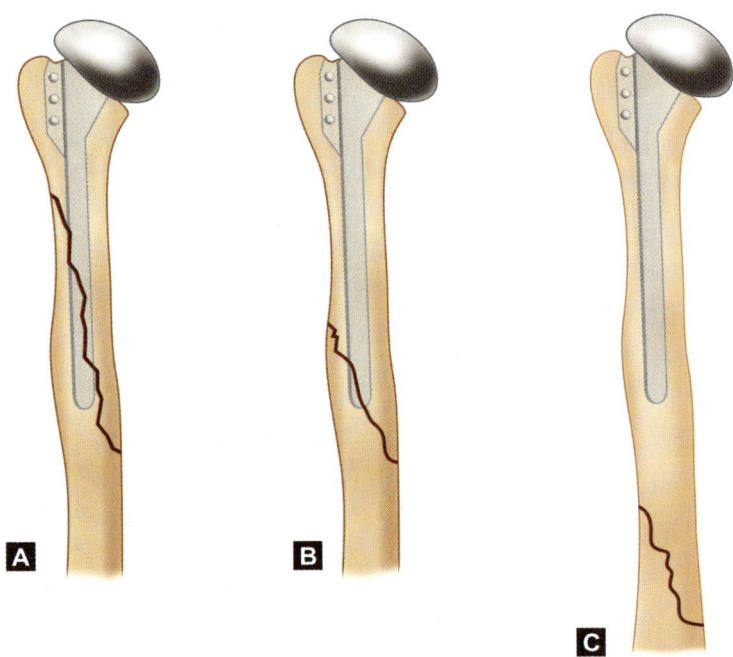

Fig. 7.8: Wright and Cofield humerus fracture after total shoulder arthroplasty.

PERIPROSTHETIC ELBOW FRACTURES

Classification (Fig. 7.9)

Type I. Periarticular/metaphyseal fracture at the level of humeral condyle/olecranon.

Type II. Fracture of the humerus or ulna in any location along the length of the prosthesis.

Type III. Fracture of the humerus/ulna distal to the prosthesis in the diaphysis.

Type IV. Fracture of the implant.

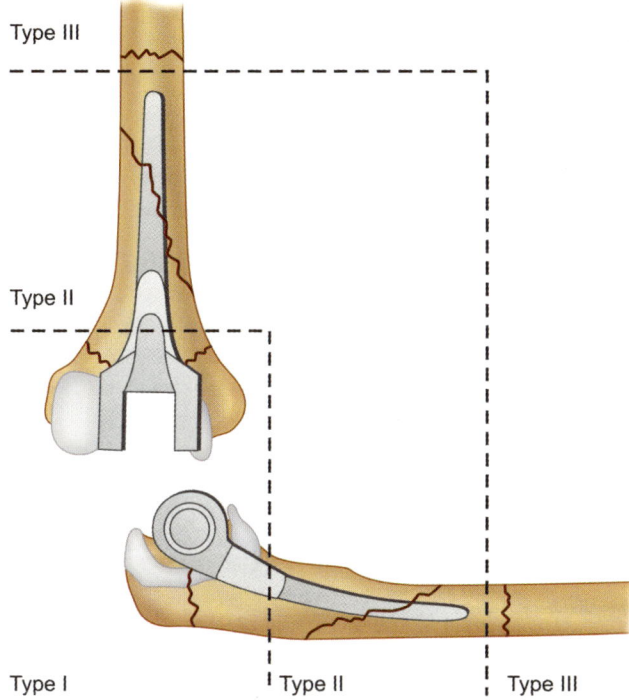

Fig. 7.9: Classification of periprosthetic elbow fractures.

Fracture Eponyms

UPPER LIMB

Mallet finger: Avulsion or rupture of extensor tendon from the base of the distal phalanx.

Jersey finger: Avulsion of flexor tendon (FDP) from base of distal phalanx.

Gamekeeper's/Skier's thumb: Avulsion of the ulnar collateral ligament at MCP joint of thumb from base of proximal phalanx.

Bennett's fracture dislocation: Oblique, displaced intra-articular fracture of the base of the first metacarpal with subluxation of the trapeziometacarpal joint such that the shaft of the first metacarpal is displaced laterally by abductor pollicis longus.

Rolando fracture: Intra-articular Y shaped fracture of the base of the first metacarpal with same but relatively less of diaphyseal displacements as a Bennett's fracture.

Boxer's fracture: Fracture through the neck of the 5th metacarpal, usually occurs in boxers.

Kaplan's dislocation: Dislocation of the MCP joint (classically of index finger).

Colles' fracture: A fracture at the cortico-cancellous junction of the distal end of the radius with dorsal tilt of distal fragment, commonly seen in postmenopausal osteoporotic females.

Smith's fracture: A fracture at the cortico-cancellous junction of the distal end of the radius with ventral tilt of distal fragment (also called reverse Colles' fracture).

Barton's fracture: Intra-articular fractures through the distal articular surface of the radius, taking a margin of radius with the carpals, displaced anteriorly or posteriorly.

Chauffeur fracture: A fracture of the styloid process of the radius.

Die punch fracture: A comminuted impacted fracture of distal radius.

Torus fracture: Special fracture pattern seen in children where a single cortex of bone is buckled inside. It is mostly seen in distal radius.

Green stick fracture: A special fracture pattern seen classically in children (due to elastic bones and a thick periosteum) where there is break in a single cortex of bone and on X-ray one finds only bending of bones.

Night stick fracture: A fracture of the shaft of ulna sustained while trying to protect from a stick blow.

Monteggia's fracture: Fracture of the proximal third of the ulna with dislocation of the radial head. Galeazzi fracture (Piedmont fracture): Fracture of the distal third of radius with subluxation of the distal radioulnar joint.

Side-swipe injury (baby car fracture): It is an elbow injury sustained when one's elbow is projecting out of a car and is side swept by another vehicle. The patient sustains fractures of the distal end of humerus with fractures of proximal ends of radius and ulna.

Nurse maid's elbow/Malgaigne's subluxation: Refers to pulled elbow which is subluxation of radial head out of the annular ligament.

Hotchkiss terrible triad of elbow injury: Comminuted fracture of the radial head, fracture of the coronoid process of ulna and posterolateral dislocation of elbow.

Luxatio erecta: Refers to inferior dislocation of shoulder.

PELVIS AND LOWER LIMB

Dashboard fracture: A fracture of posterior lip of the acetabulum, often associated with posterior dislocation of the hip (other concomitant injuries can involve femoral condyles, patella and posterior cruciate ligament).

Straddle fracture: Bilateral superior and inferior pubic rami fractures.

Pipkins fracture: Fracture of femoral head associated with posterior dislocation of hip joint.

Open book fracture: A pelvic fracture due to anteroposterior compression of pelvis where the pubic symphysis is disrupted and pelvis opens up like a book.

Malgaigne's fracture: A type of pelvis fracture due to side-to-side compression of pelvis where there is fracture of pubic rami anteriorly and sacroiliac joint or ilium posteriorly but on the same side.

Bucket handle fracture: A type of pelvis fracture due to side-to-side compression of pelvis where there is fracture of pubic rami anteriorly and sacroiliac joint or ilium posteriorly but on the opposite side.

Crescent fracture: Iliac wing fracture in pelvis that enters into SI joint.

Jumper's fracture: Transverse fracture of sacrum seen in patients who have a fall from height during a suicidal attempt. It is characterized by 'H' or 'U' shaped fracture line involving upper sacrum (S1 and S2).

Wind swept pelvis: It is a lateral compression injury of ipsilateral hemipelvis and open book or external rotation type injury of contralateral hemipelvis.

Sinding Larson disease: Avulsion injury to lower patellar pole.

Pellagrini Stieda's disease: Injury at femoral attachment of medial collateral ligament with new bone formation.

Seagond's fracture: Avulsion fracture of lateral tibial plateau with ACL injury.

Duverney fracture: Isolated iliac wing fracture.

Unresolved fracture: Neck femur fracture.

Underwear fracture: Intertrochanteric fracture.

Hoffa fracture: Fracture of the condyles of femur in coronal plane.

Bumper fracture: A fracture of the tibial plateau.

Toddler's fracture: A spiral fracture of the tibial shaft seen in toddlers due to twisting injury.

Pott's fracture: Bimalleolar ankle fracture.

Cotton's fracture: Trimalleolar ankle fracture.

Bosworth fracture: A fracture dislocation at ankle where fibula is trapped behind tibia.

Massonaie's fracture: In this an ankle fracture is associated with fracture of the neck of fibula.

Runner's fracture: Stress fracture of the distal fibula.

Pilon fracture: It is a comminuted intra-articular fracture of the distal end of tibia.

Tillaux fracture: This is avulsion of anterior tibial margin by the anterior tibiofibular ligament (Salter-Harris type III injury).

LeForte-Wagstaffe fracture: This is fibular avulsion fracture of the anterior tibiofibular ligament (counterpart of Tillaux fracture).

Aviator's fracture: Fracture of neck of talus.

Lover's fracture/Don Juan fracture: Calcaneum fracture when there is fall from height.

Chopart fracture dislocation: A fracture dislocation through intertarsal joints.

Lisfranc fracture dislocation: A fracture dislocation through tarsometatarsal joints.

Jone's fracture: Avulsion fracture of the base of the 5th metatarsal due to pull of peroneus brevis at the metaphyseo-diaphyseal junction.

Pseudo-Jones/Dancer's fracture: Avulsion fracture of the tip of 5th metatarsal.

March fracture: Stress fracture of the shafts of 2nd or 3rd metatarsal.

SPINAL FRACTURES

Jefferson's fracture: Burst fracture of the first cervical vertebra.

Whiplash injury: Cervical spine injury where sudden flexion followed by hyperextension (main damaging force) takes place.

Chance fracture: Also called seat-belt fracture, the fracture line runs horizontally through the body of the vertebra, through and through, to the posterior elements.

Burst fracture: It is a comminuted fracture of the vertebral body where fragments "burst out" in different directions often entering the canal and injuring cord.

Clay-Shoveller fracture: It is an avulsion fracture of spinous process of one or more of the lower cervical or upper thoracic vertebra (usually C7 or T1).

Hangman's fracture: It is a fracture through the pedicle and lamina of C2 vertebra, with spondylolisthesis of C2 over C3, sustained in hanging (less commonly) or in road traffic accidents (more commonly).

Chalk stick fractures: In these fractures, the fracture line is transverse to the long axis of the bone, like a broken stick of chalk. They are seen mostly in long bones in Paget's disease, osteopetrosis, ankylosing spondylitis.

Growing fractures: These are skull fractures seen mainly in infancy and early childhood characterized by progressive diastatic enlargement of the fracture line. A complication can be a cystic mass filled with CSF, called "leptomeningeal cyst".

Motorcyclist's fracture: It is a fracture of the floor of the skull. The base of the skull is divided into two halves, anterior and posterior, each moving independent of each other as if connected via hinge, hence also called "Hinge fracture".

Undertaker fracture: It is an artefact related to poor handling of the corpse characterized by subluxation of the lower cervical spine from tearing of the intervertebral disc at C6–C7 vertebral body level. It occurs due to sudden fall of the head over occipital region.

Index

A

Aitkens 109
Allman/Craig 23
Anderson and D'Alonzo classification 93
Anderson and Montesano 92
AO classification of open fractures 20
AO/OTA 1
Arazi 44
Articular
   complete 2
   partial 2

B

Bado classification 43
Bennett's fracture 49
Bohn and Durban 78
Bowers and Martin classification 91
Boyd and Griffin 67
Broberg and Morrey 40
Brumback et al classification 65
Bryan and Morrey 36
Bucket-handle injury 53
Buckle (torus) fractures 108
Burst fractures 98

C

Calcaneal fracture: Schmidt and Weiner 125
Canale and Kelly 85

Chance fractures, seat belt type injuries 99
Chopart joint 87
Colton 39
Complex 4
Cooney (universal) classification 46
Cottons fracture 83
Crescent 53

D

Dameron classification 91
Damschen 27
Danis and Weber 83
Davidson 128
Delbet classification 120
Delee classification 116
Denis classification 98, 103
Dias and Tachdjian 122
Dubberly et al 36

E

Eichenholtz and Levine classification 88
Epstein classification 63
Essex Lopresti 86
Evans 68
Evans-Jensen's 69
Extra-articular 2
Eyres and Brooks 28

F

Felix, Stuart and Hansen 129
Fernandez classification 47
Fielding 70
Fielding classification 93
Finnbogason 36
Fraser 79
Frykman classification 45

G

Galeazzi fracture 44
Ganga score 19
Garden classification 65
Garnavos 32
Gartland and Werley 44
Gotfried, Kyle, Kulkarni et al 69
Greenstick fractures 109
Gustilo-Anderson classification 18

H

Hahn-Steinthal I 36
Hahn-Steinthal II 36
Hangman's fracture 94
Harbourview 93
Hawkins classification 85, 124
Herbert and Fischer classification 48
Hohl and Moore classification 77
Hohl and Moore fracture dislocation 77
Holstein and Lewis fracture 32
Hotchkiss modification 41

I

Ideberg 28
Iliac oblique view 56
Impacted 2

J

Jackobs 36
Jahss 91
Jakob et al 114
Jensen's modification 68
Johnston modification 40

Jones
    classification 55
    fracture 91
Judet and Letournel 56
Jupiter et al 33, 43

K

Kaplan classification 51
Kilfoyle 115
King's 106
Kocher-Lorenz fragment 36
Kuhn et al 25
Kumar and Tuli's 104

L

Lauge-Hansen 83
Lenke 105
Lets et al 78
Letts classification of Monteggia's fracture 117
Levine and Edwards classification 93, 94
Lewis and Rorabeck 128
Lisfranc 89

M

Maisonneuve fracture 83
Mallet fracture 51
Mangled extrimity severity score 22
Mason 40
Mayo 38
McAfee classification 98
Mcknee et al 36
Mehne and Matta et al 33
Melone classification 46
Meyers and Mckeever classification 120
Milch 35
    classification of 114
Modified Thomas' classification 47
Modified tile 52
Monteggia equivalents 43
Monteggia fracture 41, 116
Multi-fragmentary 4
    depression of 4
Myerding grading 103
Myerson 89

N

Nash More system 106
Neer's 24, 31, 28
Nunley and Vertullo 89

O

O'Brien classification 116
O'Driscoll et al 37
Obturator oblique view 56
Ogden 111, 121
    classification of 75
Open book 53, 54

P

Patellar sleeve fracture 73
Pauwels classification 65
Peterson 112
Pilon fracture 81
Pipkin 64
Plastic deformation 108
Poland 109
Pott's
    classification 82
    fracture 83
Pseudo-Jones fracture 91
Pure depression 4
Pure split 4

Q

Quenu and Kuss 89

R

Rang 111
Ravessoud 44
Regan and Morrey 37
Riseborough and Radin 35
Risser classification 107
Robinson 24
Rockwood 25
Rolando fracture 49
Ruedi-Allgower 81

Russe classification 48
Russel-Taylor classification 71

S

Salter-Harris 109
Sanders 86
    classification of 88
Scapular index 27
Schatzker 39
Schatzker classification 76
Schenck 75
Seddon's 105
Seinsheimer classification 70
Simple 4
Smith fracture 47
Souer and Remy 86
Spondylolisthesis 103
Sprengel shoulder 107
Stewart and Milford classification 65
Supracondylar area 72
Supracondylar humerus fractures 113

T

Teisen and Hjarkbaek classification 48
Thompson and Epstein 63
Thurston-Holland fragment 110
Tillaux fracture 122
Tlics 101
Torode and Zieg 120
    classification of 55
Traynelis 92
Triplane fracture 123
Tscherne and Gotzen classification 18

V

Vancouver classification 126
Vince and Miller synostosis 119
Volar Barton 47
Volkman's fracture 83

W

Watson-Jones 121
Wedge 4

Wehbe and Schneider classification 51
Weiss et al 36
White and Panjabi 101
Wilkins and Beaty 116
Wilkins classification 116
Wiltse, Neuman and Macnab's 103
Winquist and Hansen 72

Wright and Cofield 130

Y

Young and Burgess 53

Z

Zdravkovic and Damholt 28

Reader's Note

Reader's Note

Reader's Note

Reader's Note